Praise for

Misinformed Consent

❧

"'This book eloquently and persuasively makes its case for the need for information, discussion, and counselling prior to the decision about whether to proceed with [hysterectomy]."

— B. NORMAN BARWIN, CM, M.D., FSOGC, FRCOG, FACOG, DIRECTOR, GYNECOLOGY AND INFERTILITY, THE MIDLIFE AND PMS CENTRE, OTTAWA

"Until the time when *Misinformed Consent* is required reading in every medical school, women faced with this decision should regard it as their self-defense manual in advocating for themselves."

— MICHAEL GREGER, M.D., MASSACHUSETTS, AUTHOR OF *HEART FAILURE: DIARY OF A THIRD-YEAR MEDICAL STUDENT*

"Neither fertility, zest for life, sexual functioning, nor libido can be put back, and some women are left permanently damaged by [hysterectomy]. This is the end of womanhood, and the beginning of a lifelong battle to restore a sense of well-being."

— SANDRA SIMKIN, DIRECTOR AND NATIONAL CAMPAIGN COORDINATOR, CAMPAIGN AGAINST HYSTERECTOMY AND UNNECESSARY OPERATIONS ON WOMEN, U.K., AND AUTHOR OF *THE CASE AGAINST HYSTERECTOMY* (1996)

"The most powerful tool we have for effecting transformation is knowledge. There is nothing quite as powerful as hearing the experiences of those women who have had hysterectomies. I hope the information in this book empowers women to demand better and more honest care so that we can put an end to the thousands of unnecessary hysterectomies being performed."

— MITCHELL J. LEVINE, M.D., FACOG, CHIEF OF THE DEPARTMENT OF OBSTETRICS AND GYNECOLOGY AT THE DEACONESS WALTHAM HOSPITAL IN WALTHAM, MASSACHUSETTS, AND DIRECTOR OF THE WOMEN CARE ORGANIZATION

"The truth about the potentially devastating side effects of medical procedures and drugs should come from medical professionals. Instead, so much of the vital information comes from survivors like Lise Cloutier-Steele, who possess the courage to write about medicine's often-tragic results because they themselves learned too late about the dark side of medicine."

— TONDA R. BIAN, INVESTIGATIVE JOURNALIST, FLORIDA, AUTHOR OF
THE DRUG LORDS: AMERICA'S PHARMACEUTICAL CARTEL (1997)

"It is still difficult to persuade some medical students that reproductive-associated organs may contribute to health and well-being unrelated to childbearing. This book should be required reading for any prospective hysterectomy patient."

— THE LATE MARIE M. CASSIDY, PH.D., DSC, CITIZENS FOR
RESPONSIBLE CARE AND RESEARCH, NEW YORK

"*Misinformed Consent* is a reminder to medical professionals that good communication is the foundation of the patient-doctor relationship, and that above all else, they should do no harm."

— BARBARA A. YEATS, M.D., CCFP, OTTAWA

"This is a work born of pain . . . that may help to prevent more suffering."

— AVIS FAVARO, MEDICAL CORRESPONDENT, CTV TELEVISION NETWORK, TORONTO

"*Misinformed Consent* is an extraordinary source of information! Every woman who reads this book will be better prepared to face doctors, not just gynecologists, but specialists from all other medical domains."

— ALICE RÉGNIER, RN, MONTRÉAL

"*Misinformed Consent* is a carefully reasoned analysis and chilling exposé of the insidious betrayal of women who are hysterectomized. After all the research and writing I have done on world-wide atrocities against women under patriarchy, this book still manages to inform and shock me."

— MARY DALY, PH.D., MASSACHUSETTS, AUTHOR OF BEYOND GOD
THE FATHER, GYN/ECOLOGY: THE METAETHICS OF RADICAL FEMINISM
AND QUINTESSENCE: REALIZING THE ARCHAIC FUTURE

"Think of how men would respond if their doctors wanted to remove their testicles and prostate glands once they had all the children they wanted, and then put them on synthetic testosterone drugs. Removing a woman's ovaries is no less a violation and has equally devastating consequences."

— JOHN R. LEE, M.D., CALIFORNIA, AUTHOR OF
WHAT YOUR DOCTOR MAY NOT TELL YOU ABOUT MENOPAUSE

"*Misinformed Consent* is a book that should be read by every woman contemplating a hysterectomy, by every medical student and physician, [and by] husbands, lovers, and friends of women contemplating a hysterectomy."

— RUTH HARRIET JACOBS, PH.D., AUTHOR OF *BE AN OUTRAGEOUS OLDER WOMAN*

"We do not know enough about the human variation in the body's delicate hormonal rhythms to surgically excise the organs where they originate without great caution and more information. We need research in this area to better understand the hormonal roots of our joys, sexual drives, pleasures, and pains. The stories in this book should motivate researchers to look for those roots."

— DUANE F. STROMAN, PH.D., PENNSYLVANIA, AUTHOR OF *THE MEDICAL
ESTABLISHMENT AND SOCIAL RESPONSIBILITY* (1976), *QUICK KNIFE: UNNECESSARY
SURGERY U.S.A.* (1979), AND *MENTAL RETARDATION IN SOCIAL CONTEXT* (1989)

"*Misinformed Consent* is a sobering call to women, and the men who love them, to examine carefully a prescription for hysterectomy. If you are considering hysterectomy . . . don't let anyone fool you into believing that the hormones you lose can be replaced."

— WINNIFRED B. CUTLER, PH.D., FOUNDER AND PRESIDENT, ATHENA INSTITUTE,
PENNSYLVANIA, AND AUTHOR OF SEVERAL BOOKS, INCLUDING
HYSTERECTOMY BEFORE AND AFTER AND *MENOPAUSE:
A GUIDE FOR WOMEN AND THE MEN WHO LOVE THEM*

"*Misinformed Consent* confirms my opinion that the medical profession does not really know how to treat women."

— MEL ALTER, BSCPHM, LPH, FACA, PHARMACIST, MONTRÉAL

"This book documents unnecessary surgery, incompetently perpetrated, with devastating results on the women and their families."

— EILEEN MARIE WAYNE, M.D., ILLINOIS, INFORMEDCONSENT.ORG

"The personal and poignant accounts found in *Misinformed Consent* demonstrate how the present autopilot of so-called informed consent must be corrected. As a family physician and Member of Parliament, it is distressing to me that women are clearly being subjected to unnecessary and sometimes debilitating surgery. This book is extremely important, not only in elucidating the problem, but also in providing practical suggestions for the real solution — empowerment."

— CAROLYN BENNETT, M.D., MEMBER OF PARLIAMENT, HOUSE OF COMMONS, OTTAWA

"Every doctor should read this book before recommending a hysterectomy. Women need all the information available. We don't need to be 'protected' from the facts."

— FAY CAMPBELL, MSEd, ASSOCIATE DIRECTOR,
ENDOMETRIOSIS ASSOCIATION, WISCONSIN

"The powerful language, the compelling stories, the true effects of life after hysterectomy make this book a must-read for every woman and a wake-up call to medical professionals."

— CHARLES B. INLANDER, PRESIDENT, PEOPLE'S MEDICAL SOCIETY, PENNSYLVANIA

"This book deserves the attention of any woman making a major decision about her health — straight talk by women for women, and a networking system to voice fears and questions about your health."

— AGNES HERON, PRESIDENT OF WOMENTLC.COM, FLORIDA, AND
RADIO TALK-SHOW HOST ON WOMEN'S HEALTH

"Lise Cloutier-Steele and the other contributors to this volume have very courageously broken the myths and silence surrounding hysterectomy and its aftermath. A definite must-read for all women who are faced with this life-altering decision."

— G. ASHA, NEUROSCIENTIST, INDIA

"Incredible, heart-breaking true stories all women will want to read and share."
— SONDRA FOREST, M.S.W., A.C.S.W., C.S.W., CAC1
CLINICAL SOCIAL WORKER, FAMILY SERVICE, INC., DEARBORN, MICHIGAN

"Give this book to any friend before she has a hysterectomy. It is a vivid reminder that we must take charge of our own medical care. There are many caring, knowledgeable and careful doctors who can be trusted, and there are also doctors who can't. Unfortunately, your failure to investigate may be a life-changing event. On a personal note, how lucky we all are to have sources like Oprah, Donahue and the news media to alert us to new developments in medicine!"
— MARJORIE BEKAERT THOMAS, PRESIDENT, IVANHOE BROADCAST NEWS, FLORIDA

"The brave, beleagured women who tell their stories in *Misinformed Consent* provide us with vivid proof that most women and most physicians remain woefully ignorant about the alternatives to and the consequences of unnecessary hysterectomy. In order to ensure that we and our physicians become better informed, this poignant book begins with a strong demand for change and ends with a comprehensive list of resources that help women better protect themselves."
— JANE PINCUS, CO-AUTHOR OF *OUR BODIES, OURSELVES FOR THE NEW CENTURY*
CO-FOUNDER OF THE BOSTON WOMEN'S HEALTH BOOK COLLECTIVE

"This book is a must, before any woman gives consent to a hysterectomy or oophorectomy. Get informed first and learn about the alternatives to avoid surgery."
— PETE HUESEMAN, R.PH.,P.D., CONSULTANT PHARMACIST, ST. LOUIS, MISSOURI
WWW. BPHARMACYSOLUTIONS.COM

"I feel sad that this work is needed, but glad that it was done so well."
— PETER R. MANSFIELD, M.D.
DEPARTMENT OF GENERAL PRACTICE, UNIVERSITY OF ADELAIDE, AUSTRALIA
DIRECTOR, HEALTHY SKEPTICISM, WWW.HEALTHYSKEPTICISM.ORG

Misinformed Consent

Women's Stories about
Unnecessary Hysterectomy

LISE CLOUTIER-STEELE

FOREWORD BY STANLEY T. WEST, M.D.
OVERVIEW BY MARY ANNE WYATT

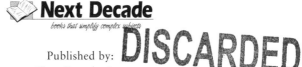

Next Decade
books that simply complex subjects

Published by:
Next Decade, Inc.
39 Old Farmstead Road
Chester, New Jersey 07930-2702
www.nextdecade.com

Published by:
Next Decade, Inc.
39 Old Farmstead Road
Chester, New Jersey 07930-2732 USA
www.nextdecade.com

Library of Congress Cataloging-in-Publication Data

Cloutier-Steele, Lise.
  Misinformed consent : women's stories about unnecessary hysterectomy / Lise Cloutier-Steele ; foreword by Stanley T. West ; overview by Mary Anne Wyatt.
     p. cm.
  ISBN 0-9700908-6-2 (pbk. : alk. paper)
  1. Hysterectomy--Popular works. 2. Surgery, Unnecessary--Popular works. I. Title.
  RG391 .C62 2003
  618.1'453--dc21

                                        2002152481

To protect their privacy, some of the contributors' names and identifying characteristics have been changed.

Cover design: Paul A. Richer
Text design: Tannice Goddard
Typesetting: Kinetics Design

$16.95 Softcover

Disclaimer

The purpose of this book is to tell the stories of several women who underwent unnecessary hysterectomy. It is presented with the understanding that the publisher and author are not engaged in rendering medical advice or other professional services in this book. When medical or other expert assistance is required, the services of a competent professional should be sought.

This manual was not written to provide all the information that is available to the author/and or publisher, but to complement, amplify and supplement other texts and available information. While every effort has been made to ensure that this book is as complete and accurate as possible, there may be mistakes, either typographical or in content. Therefore, this text should be used as a general guide only, and not as the ultimate source of hysterectomy and alternative information. Furthermore, this book contains current information only up to the printing date.

Information herein was obtained from various sources whose accuracy is not guaranteed. Opinions expressed and information are subject to change without notice.

The author and Next Decade, Inc. shall not be held liable, nor be responsible to any person or entity with respect to any loss or damage caused, or alleged to be caused, directly or indirectly by the information contained in this book.

If you do not wish to be bound by the above, you may return this book to the publisher for a full refund.

To my husband, Paul, for loving me always,
even on the dark days.

And to the memory of Marie Mullaney Cassidy, Ph.D., DSc

Dr. Cassidy was a founding member and officer of CIRCARE (Citizens for Responsible Care and Research), New York, and one of the longest-serving professors at the George Washington University Medical Center. She was known for her commitment to causes that aimed to improve the lives of the less fortunate. Dr. Cassidy was devoted to CIRCARE's mission to improve ethical standards in research that involves people, and as a leader in the feminist movement, she mentored other women in leadership roles.

Contents

Acknowledgements

*T*his work was meant to be. I am very appreciative of the courage displayed by all the contributors to this book. I know it wasn't easy for some of you, yet your submissions fell into *Misinformed Consent* like the pieces of a puzzle — a perfect fit.

I am especially grateful to you, Faith, for your encouragement from the time I thought of the idea for this publication until the very end. Thank you, Beth, for throwing me a lifeline when I needed one. This book is in fact an homage to all your good work on behalf of hysterectomized women around the world. Thanks for your cheerful messages, Jeannah; they brought a smile to my lips every time.

Without you, Mary Anne, this book could never be. Knowing about your pain and the physical difficulties you face each day, I will always be in your debt for your generous contributions to this work, your support, and, most of all, your friendship.

I remain indebted to you as well, Elizabeth, for your vote of confidence. It meant a lot to me. I am equally grateful to you, Dawn, for your ongoing encouragement and your many supportive e-mails.

To my Canadian connections — Tracee, Amber, Carol, and Pat — many thanks for your friendship. It gives me a great feeling knowing that we will never be alone again.

Though we are an ocean apart, Angela, the closeness we shared over the past four years is just the beginning. And thank you, Eve, for being the woman that you are.

You were my number-one fan and cheering section, Ellen. You gave me strength and laughter, and you gave me the best that you can give — yourself.

To Gayle, my sincere thanks for your courage. Phoebe, thank you for your support and your determination to make a difference for others. Many thanks to Roberta, Penny, LaShonda and Chere for meeting my very tight deadline, and making the revised edition more complete.

I am grateful to David Elver for working with me on this important project. His assistance in polishing the manuscript proved invaluable when it came time to introduce the book proposal to publishers.

My heartfelt thanks go out to Dr. Stanley T. West for his wonderful critique and for making time to write the excellent foreword to this book (I knew it would be perfect). A special thank you to Montreal-based compounding pharmacist Mel Alter, who provided an informative overview of natural hormone replacement therapy for the introduction. To all the experts who reviewed this work — Sandra Simkin of the U.K.; Tonda R. Bian and Agnes Heron of Florida; Alice Régnier of Montréal; Avis Favaro of Toronto; Doctors Carolyn Bennett, Barbara A. Yeats, and B. Norman Barwin of Ottawa; Fay Campbell of Wisconsin; Doctors Ruth Harriet Jacobs, Michael Greger, Mitchell J. Levine, and Mary Daly of Massachusetts; Dr. Eileen Marie Wayne of Illinois; Dr. John R. Lee of California; the late Dr. Marie Cassidy of Washington, D.C.; Charles B. Inlander, Doctors Winnifred B. Cutler, and Duane F. Stroman of Pennsylvania; and neuroscientist G. Asha of India — your endorsement of this project gives hysterectomized women a better chance to be understood.

One last person deserves my thanks and gratitude: Susan Goldberg. Her passion about the issue of unnecessary hysterectomy and her flair for editing added great value to this project. I know I speak for all the contributors when I say that it was a pleasure to have worked with you.

To all the experts who reviewed this work — Sandra Simkin of the U.K.; Tonda R. Bian and Agnes Heron, and Marjorie Bekaert Thomas of Florida; Alice Régnier of Montréal; Avis Favaro of Toronto; Doctors Carolyn Bennett, Barbara A. Yeats, and B. Norman Barwin of Ottawa; Fay Campbell of Wisconsin; Sondra Forest of Michigan; Jane Pincus and Doctors Ruth Harriet Jacobs, Michael Greger, Mitchell J. Levine, and Mary Daly of Massachusetts; Dr. Eileen Marie Wayne of Illinois; Dr. John R. Lee of California; the late Dr. Marie Cassidy of Washington, D.C.; Charles B. Inlander, Doctors Winnifred B. Cutler, and Duane F. Stroman of Pennsylvania; Pete Hueseman of Missouri; Dr. Peter R. Mansfield of Australia and neuroscientist G. Asha of India — your endorsement of this project gives hysterectomized women a better chance to be understood.

PART I

Introduction

"Both abundance and lack exist simultaneously in our lives, as parallel realities. It is always our conscious choice which secret garden we will tend . . . when we choose not to focus on what is missing from our lives, but are grateful for the abundance that's present — love, health, family, friends, work, the joys of nature and personal pursuits that bring us pleasure — the wasteland of illusion falls away and we experience Heaven on earth."

— SARAH BAN BREATHNACH

"Women are not entirely wrong when they reject the rules of life prescribed for the world, for they were established by men only, without their consent."

— MICHEL EYQUEM DE MONTAIGNE, 1588

"My concern is that in their haste to carry out a procedure such as hysterectomy, perhaps gynecologists do not spend enough time discussing the implications of surgery and the potential effect on quality of life."

— ALVIN PETTLE, M.D., FRCS(C), 2000

Foreword

❧

Stanley T. West, M.D., FACOG

When I was in medical school, a prominent surgeon named George Crille spoke to us about his results in the management of breast cancer. He presented his statistics, which showed that simple mastectomy, or surgical removal of the breast, yielded the same results as the more radical and disfiguring Halstead technique, which involved removing not only the entire breast, but the surrounding tissues, muscles in the chest wall, and lymph nodes as well.

"Why should we disfigure women?" he asked. Doctors didn't need to perform radical mastectomies, he told us; they often left women depressed and with one arm swollen.

Well, Dr. Crille was roundly condemned. After all, what did women know? What did their opinions or emotions matter? Who cared what they looked like after surgery? Women weren't doctors. Besides, if the medical profession took "hysterical" women's opinions into account, they would just opt for the latest craze. On and on went the debate. Not once, however, were the statistics challenged. Nor was consideration of the operation's effect on patients mentioned.

Today, radical mastectomy is rarely performed. Even simple mastectomy has given way to lumpectomy, the removal of only the tumour, as the new surgical "gold standard." Did the medical profession suddenly achieve an epiphany? Of course not. Rather, women — empowered by knowledge — stated simply that they would no longer allow a disfiguring operation to be performed when they could undergo an equally successful surgery without the negative consequences. Doctors suddenly found that, if they wished to remain in practice, they needed to listen to their patients. What a radical idea!

After medical school, I trained in gynecology and infertility. A number of my patients had fibroid tumours that prevented them from getting pregnant. I began reading about myomectomy, the surgical removal of fibroids while leaving the uterus and ovaries intact. When I inquired about the procedure, my colleagues asked why in the world I wanted to do such a difficult surgery when I could just perform a hysterectomy to remove the entire uterus. "Just take it out," I was told.

When I mentioned that women experienced all kinds of problems following hysterectomy, I was told, "Well, you know that females are basically hysterical." Fortunately, articles began appearing in peer journals that substantiated the problems created by hysterectomy. Books for the lay public began to appear, and these gave women the knowledge to do battle with their doctors and to demand alternatives to hysterectomy.

However, most of the articles and books were written by those of us in the medical profession who had experienced the downside of hysterectomy only second-hand. Lise Cloutier-Steele has brought together a collection of women's personal experiences that document first-hand the problems with hysterectomy. While there will continue to be physicians who steadfastly maintain that hysterectomy is an uncomplicated procedure, books like *Misinformed Consent* that document why it is not will eventually win out.

When Lise asked me to write the foreword, I eagerly accepted. Like George Crille, I am convinced that women will prevail and force the medical profession to listen. Lise's book hammers yet another nail into the coffin of the myth that a woman does not need her uterus.

Hysterectomy:
Its Prevalence, Rationale,
and Aftereffects

❦

*A*s I contemplate my much larger face in the mirror, I wonder if there will ever be a time when I can be more accepting of the new me. I know the change in my weight is directly linked to the hysterectomy I had in October 1991 and to the estrogen replacement therapy I have been on ever since. The extra weight will likely never come off, and yet I continue with diet programs, hoping that all the plump areas will one day disappear.

Don't ask me where my head was when I agreed to the surgical removal of my reproductive organs — I just don't know. At the age of thirty-eight, I am embarrassed to say, I was clueless about the role my reproductive organs played beyond their childbearing capability. When I compare the symptoms I had before surgery to the complications that surfaced after my hysterectomy, I realize that I am no further ahead. In fact, my quality of life has taken a nosedive.

It wasn't until January 1998, when I saw a television program on sexual desire, that I made the connection between my extinguished libido and my hysterectomy. The overload of information from that program was mind-boggling. Many of the young women interviewed on the show discussed their loss of sexual desire and the effect of this loss on their relationships. I felt numb when one guest spoke about her depression and her loss of sexual drive and sensation following her hysterectomy, and how she had not felt like a whole woman since.

She was talking about me.

I felt relieved, sad, and angry all at once. It wasn't the first time I had experienced a mixed bag of emotions; I ride an emotional roller coaster almost every day. But this time the feelings were much more intense, and they made me realize that I had a lot of work to do. Little did I know that my research into the effects of hysterectomy would lead me to so many other women just like me, and eventually to this book.

These new connections quickly translated into ongoing support, encouragement, and friendships with very special women whose hysterectomy stories had to be told. I wanted women facing the possibility of hysterectomy to be afforded a glimpse into the lives of women who had been through the procedure — and who were willing to share their innermost secrets — in the hope of sparing others from an irreversible, and often unnecessary, surgery. This book is about women hoping to help other women.

As the contributions poured in, and as I read each story for the first time, I was astounded, both at the wealth of information these women had provided and at the many parallels between their experiences and my own. I wasn't alone after all. I immediately felt a strong bond with all the contributors who, like me, are determined to find their way back to better health.

We know that many women who have hysterectomies feel absolutely wonderful afterwards. But large numbers of women have had markedly negative experiences with hysterectomy, and growing numbers of hysterectomized women are now speaking out about the ill effects of this drastic surgery. It may well be that those glowing reports on the positive outcomes of hysterectomies are not entirely accurate. Very little information is available about the outcome of surgery from the patient's perspective.[1] Without more and better research into the long-term effects hysterectomy and female castration, women cannot truly give informed consent to this operation.

In the past, women typically kept quiet about personal health-related issues such as sexual dysfunction, mood swings, menstrual problems, and depression. I know my mother would have had tremendous difficulty discussing these subjects with any doctor. In her day, it was simply not done. Today's women are more open. I feel strongly that discussing the potential negative effects of hysterectomy is key to slowing the alarming rate at which this surgical procedure is performed.

In North America, hysterectomy appears to have been one of the most popular — and often unnecessary — surgical procedures of the 1990s and now into the new millennium. In Canada alone, for instance, sixty-two thousand hysterectomies are performed each year. This represents one of the highest rates in the world, second only to the United States, where roughly seven hundred thousand are performed annually, and almost double the rate of most European countries. In fact, 37 percent of Canadian women will have had a hysterectomy by the age of sixty. By that same age, one in every three women in the United States has had a hysterectomy; by age sixty-five, the proportion increases to one out of two. Most of these procedures — as many as 90 percent — are elective. And, argues Dr. Stanley West, author of *The Hysterectomy Hoax*, nine out of ten hysterectomies are unnecessary.

In the province of Ontario, where I live, hysterectomy is the most commonly performed surgical procedure. More than twenty thousand were performed in 1994–95 alone. The choice of hysterectomy may coincide more with the inclinations and surgical abilities of local gynecologists than with medical imperatives; there seems to be little rhyme or reason in how doctors prescribe and perform this often life-altering operation. According to the Toronto Institute for Clinical Evaluative

---

1 A study by Charles J. Wright, M.D., MSc, FRCS (C, E.Ed), on the large-scale outcomes of six surgical procedures in western Canada, including hysterectomy, was released in May 2001. Dr. Wright is a former surgeon and the director of the Centre for Clinical Epidemiology and Evaluation at Vancouver Hospital and Health Sciences Centre.

Sciences (ICES), the rate of hysterectomy per region ranges from 274 to 797 per 100,000 women.[2] Not surprisingly, in early 1998, the Ontario Medical Association published a report (not circulated to the public) stating that too many hysterectomies were being performed in Ontario.

But a new report addressing the issue of the overuse of hysterectomy in Canada *was* made public in June 2002. It confirmed that Canada's situation is similar to that of the United States. Dr. Donna Stewart, professor at the University of Toronto and chair of Women's Health at the University Health Network, led the expert panel on hysterectomy practices in Ontario. A complete copy of the panel's report can be viewed at www.ontariowomenscouncil.on.ca. (See Medical Resources in Part III for more information on the Ontario Women's Council.)

According to Dr. Stewart, there are many factors contributing to the high rate of hysterectomy. For instance, many doctors are unwilling to explore other less invasive treatments with their patients. This is an unfortunate situation in itself, because if a woman is not offered less drastic options, she is not given the opportunity to make an informed choice.

Education and social class are two other important factors, and Dr. Stewart's report shows that the hysterectomy rate is highest in poor, rural regions where the level of education is low. Similarly in the U.S., the hysterectomy rate is highest in the southern states. And surprisingly, some women view hysterectomy as a permanent solution for birth control, while others feel it's the "thing to do", because it's what their mothers and sisters did before them. In any case, none of the above explanations justify a prolongation of the current situation of unnecessary surgeries performed on female patients, but all confirm the need for greater education efforts to help women and their doctors discuss less invasive alternatives to hysterectomy.

These facts are all the more disturbing when we consider that the substantial majority of hysterectomies are very likely unnecessary. Along

---

2 Cohen, M.M., and W. Young. "Hysterectomy, Variations in Selected Surgical Procedures and Medical Diagnoses by Year and Region." *Patterns of Health Care in Ontario: The ICES Practice Atlas*. Goel W. Williams, J.I., G.M. Anderson, P. Blackstein-Hirsch, C. Fooks, and C.D. Naylor, ed. 2nd ed. (Ottawa: Canadian Medical Association, 1996), 116, 119.

with Dr. West, Sandra Simkin, author of *The Case Against Hysterectomy*, argues that 90 percent of hysterectomies are unwarranted and do not effectively treat the conditions for which they are prescribed. Surgically excising the uterus, Fallopian tubes, cervix, and/or ovaries is necessary only if cancer has been detected in one of these organs. Often, however, women are convinced to surrender their healthy reproductive organs "just in case" they might one day become cancerous. The logic of this approach is fundamentally flawed, and reveals how little the medical profession seems to value women's reproductive organs. Doctors rarely, if ever, urge men to surgically excise healthy testicles "just in case" they might one day become cancerous! As you will read in my personal story, my family physician used this scare tactic, among others, to get me to agree to a hysterectomy. It worked.

Exploring Other Options

Hysterectomy is an irreversible procedure. I cannot emphasize enough the importance of exploring other treatment options before considering this extreme surgery. It should be regarded as a last resort only, especially if cancer has not been detected. Many alternative therapies are available to treat the conditions for which hysterectomy is often indicated.

For instance, to investigate women's common complaints of painful menses, excessive menstrual bleeding, or chronic pelvic pain, many doctors prescribe dilation and curettage (D&C), a procedure in which the cervix is dilated and the lining of the uterus is scraped away. Dilation and curettage can aid doctors in assessing the condition of the endometrium, or lining of the uterus. Often, two or three D&Cs can be performed before the word "hysterectomy" need even be mentioned.

Microwave endometrial ablation (MEA) is a newer, less invasive procedure to treat heavy bleeding from menstruation. A surgeon inserts an applicator into the uterus to burn the uterine lining with low-power microwaves. Following this procedure, monthly periods are either eliminated or the flow is considerably reduced. (Since it can result in infertility, this procedure is recommended only for women who don't want any, or any more, children.)

Laparoscopy is another minimally invasive surgical technique, which uses a fibre-optic camera inserted through a small incision. It can be an effective tool for identifying and treating chronic pelvic pain.

Hysterectomy is routinely recommended to treat uterine fibroids and endometriosis, two conditions for which viable alternative procedures are available. Much progress has been made in alternative treatments of these conditions over the past twenty years. If these new procedures can minimize negative outcomes for women's bodies, minds, and souls, doctors have an obligation to try every possible treatment available before recommending hysterectomy.

Uterine Fibroids

Fibroids, or *leiomyoma uteri*, are benign (non-cancerous) tumours made of muscle tissue that form in the uterine wall. Fibroid removal is the most common reason for hysterectomies in the United States, and accounts for about 30 percent (or two hundred thousand operations a year) of all such procedures performed in that country. There are also numerous procedures to treat fibroids directly *without* removal of the uterus.

Nobody knows why fibroids develop, although we do know that estrogen can trigger their formation and growth. Fibroids are generally harmless; approximately 40 percent of women of childbearing age have at least one fibroid tumour, and most don't even know it's there.

In some women, however, fibroid tumours grow large enough to interfere with reproductive and pelvic function. Women with large fibroids can experience abdominal or lower back pain, urinary problems such as frequent urination, incontinence, or repeated urinary tract infections, and heavy menstrual flow. Some women report labour-like pain, tenderness, or aching in the uterus, as well as painful intercourse. Fibroids may interfere with a woman's ability to conceive or to successfully complete a pregnancy.

Therapies to treat uterine fibroids include myomectomy (removal of the fibroids only, *not* the entire uterus); uterine artery embolization (UAE), which cuts off the blood supply to the fibroids, causing them to shrink and die; and myolysis, which involves using drugs to shrink the fibroids, laser surgery to pierce them, and electrical charges to destroy the blood vessels that feed them. Cryomyolysis uses the very low temperature of liquid nitrogen to literally freeze fibroids to death.

Many doctors don't have the surgical skills to perform operations such as myomectomy, which can be considerably more difficult than a hysterectomy. Sadly, a gynecologist's recommendations may have more to do with his or her own skills and comfort level than with the best course of treatment for the patient. Unfortunately, *money may also play a role in some doctors' recommendations for treatment of fibroids*. For example, interventional radiologists (IRs), not gynecologists, perform UAE, so gynecologists lose surgical fees when they refer a patient to an IR. It is crucial that women with problematic fibroids understand that hysterectomy is neither the only nor necessarily the best option for treating this condition.

Endometriosis

Endometriosis remains a mysterious disease. According to many experts, its cause is unknown, yet it afflicts millions. Endometriosis occurs when tissue that normally lines the uterus migrates out of that organ into — and occasionally beyond — the pelvic cavity. It can implant itself on other organs and in the lining of the pelvic cavity, where it continues to bleed each month. It can cause irregular bleeding, painful menses, and cramping. Endometriosis plagues an estimated 15 percent of women. For women who are estrogen-deficient, it tends to diminish with menopause. If the disease is not addressed, the endometrial implants can fuse together a woman's internal organs. Endometriosis can also result in infertility. (For further information on endometriosis, see Publications of Interest in Part III.)

There appears to be extensive debate in the medical community as to whether endometriosis should be treated with hysterectomy and oophorectomy (surgical removal of the ovaries). However, remarkable new drugs, as well as some very sophisticated surgical techniques, says Dr. Stanley West, "have made it possible to eradicate endometrial implants and associated adhesions simply and quickly."[3]

Premenstrual Syndrome (PMS)

I have talked to and corresponded with many women who have considered hysterectomy in the hope that it would cure them of the symptoms of premenstrual syndrome. To all these women I stress that PMS is a condition for which a hysterectomy is absolutely *not* justifiable. Castration is simply not a reasonable treatment for mood swings and other PMS symptoms.

Dr. Katharina Dalton, the foremost authority on PMS research and its treatment, and author of *Once a Month*, writes that hysterectomy is not the answer for women suffering from premenstrual syndrome, however severe their symptoms may be. According to Dalton, the sudden changes brought on by surgical menopause affect only the ovaries and the uterus, leaving the menstrual clock in the brain intact. This means that those who suffer from premenstrual syndrome prior to hysterectomy will continue to see their symptoms return on a cyclical basis.

Hormone therapy, nutritional supplements, and exercise often prove to be very effective methods of treatment for PMS. *Once a Month* includes chapters on what your doctor can do to help you with PMS symptoms, what you can do to help yourself, and a list of resources and PMS clinics and support groups in the United States. (See Publications of Interest in Part III for further information on this book.)

Potential Side Effects

Hysterectomy and oophorectomy are not mild procedures with no aftereffects. These surgeries have a profound impact on a woman's well-being. Doctors have traditionally downplayed the risks involved in the

---

3 West, Stanley, with Paula Dranov. *The Hysterectomy Hoax*. (New Jersey, Next Decade, Inc., 2002), 115.

operation and its aftereffects, argue Simkin and other researchers, such as Dr. Judith Reichman, author of *I'm Too Young to Get Old.*

Like any other invasive surgery, hysterectomy and oophorectomy carry risks that include pain and scarring, internal bleeding, long recovery periods, complications, surgical incompetence, reactions to anesthetic, and, in the worst scenario, death.

In addition to general surgical risks, hysterectomy and oophorectomy are associated with a number of specific side effects that range from mild to severe. "Hysterectomized women," writes Dr. Lois Jovanovic in *A Woman Doctor's Guide to Menopause*, "reportedly suffer far more severe menopausal symptoms than those who lose ovarian function gradually."[4] These symptoms can include allergies, arthritis, bowel dysfunction, bloating, cardiovascular disease, cyclic edema, depression, loss of normal body-fat pads, gallstones, generalized fatigue, hot flashes, incontinence, insomnia, masculinization, memory loss, chronic migraines, loss of orgasm, osteoporosis, severe PMS, loss of sexual desire and drive, rapid aging of the skin, thyroid dysfunction, and weight gain (sometimes called "Buddha belly").

The stories in this book will provide insight into almost all the difficulties linked with hysterectomy. However, a number of symptoms common to many hysterectomized women merit special mention here.

Flushing and Night Sweats

The flush (or hot flash) is the most common aftereffect of surgical menopause, and is thought to be caused by estrogen deficiency. Even though many hysterectomized women take estrogen supplements, they can still flush. For some, it can take years to find the right mix of supplements to help keep the flushes under control.

Ask any woman who lives with this difficulty, and she will tell you that flushing is *very* uncomfortable. I can flush up to three or four times an hour. The episodes are accompanied by an increased heartbeat that

---

4 Jovanovic, Lois, with Suzanne LeVert. *A Woman Doctor's Guide to Menopause.* (New York: Hyperion, 1993).

makes me anxious. The surge of heat intensifies from the middle of my body to the top of my head. My face and neck turn red and I perspire, which is frustrating and, at times, embarrassing. The flush eventually reaches a peak, after which I feel a slow release of the intense heat.

Night sweats are the nighttime version of the flush. Too many night sweats can severely disrupt a woman's sleep, leaving her fatigued, moody, and irritable.

Depression

As early as 1968, medical researchers noted that "hysterectomy seemed to be associated with more post-operative depression than other forms of surgery."[5] Many subsequent studies have documented the same phenomenon. Still, many well-meaning physicians are not aware of the documented relationship between hysterectomy and depression, says Dr. Winnifred Cutler: "Why? Because the physicians who do the surgery or who recommend the surgery tend not to follow the cases of these women two or three years after their surgery, and the depression usually begins after the last post surgical check-up."[6]

Post-hysterectomy depression is most likely to occur in women who

- are under forty years old at the time of the operation,
- have a previous history of depression, especially postnatal depression,
- had no gynecological abnormality detected at operation,
- have a history of marital disruption, and
- have had previous sterilization operations, such as tubal ligation.[7]

I fit into all five categories listed above, so perhaps it is not surprising that depression is a health problem that I contend with to this day. Most of the mechanisms I used to cope with depression in the past no longer

---

5 Barker, M.G., "Psychiatric Illness After Hysterectomy," *Br Med J* 2 (1968), 91–95.
6 Cutler, Winnifred B. *Hysterectomy Before and After: A Comprehensive Guide to Preventing, Preparing for, and Maximizing Health After Hysterectomy*. (New York: HarperCollins, 1989), 253.
7 Dalton, Katharina. *Once a Month*. (Great Britain: Fontana Paperbacks, 1978), 225.

serve me well. Women who suffer from this disorder should know that all a hysterectomy does is stop menstrual flow. It is not a cure for depression.

Decreased Libido

Decreased libido, or sex drive, is one of the most devastating consequences of hysterectomy, and can seriously hinder a woman's sexual and emotional well-being. As early as 1975, Dr. Wulf H. Utian reported a "high incidence of decreased or absent libido in all groups of patients having undergone the operation of hysterectomy, irrespective of whether the ovaries had been conserved."[8]

Further studies concur with Dr. Utian's findings. Sandra Simkin, for example, reported in 1996 that "research carried out in the United States has revealed that all hysterectomy patients experience a high incidence of decreased or absent libido, whether or not their ovaries are retained, and that estrogen replacement does not restore libido following hysterectomy, although it does counteract vaginal dryness and atrophy, and reduces menopausal symptoms."[9]

I wonder to this day why no one discussed this side effect with me before my surgery. Until then, I had enjoyed a perfectly healthy sex life, a fact that was clearly irrelevant to the physicians involved in my hysterectomy. A woman's libido is as important as her blood pressure, says Dr. Judith Reichman. No woman should have to live without sexual desire.

Perforations and Sexual Dysfunction

A hysterectomy is a very complicated surgical procedure that requires great skill in order to avoid nerve damage and accidental perforations. When gynecologists clamp and cut during surgery, they can potentially damage nerves that affect sexual function. Hysterectomized women

---

8 Utian, Wulf H., "Effect of Hysterectomy, Oophorectomy and Estrogen Therapy on Libido," *Int J Obstet Gyn* 13 (1975), 97–100.

9 Simkin, Sandra. *The Case Against Hysterectomy*. (London: Pandora, An Imprint of HarperCollins, 1996), 33.

often report perforated bowels and punctured bladders. The subsequent repairs can result in further scars and adhesions (internal scar tissue) that impinge on a woman's quality of life as well as her sexual response.

Hysterectomy can leave a woman with a shortened vagina, making penetrative sex difficult or impossible. This complication occurs most frequently when surgeons remove the cervix (the narrow lower part of the uterus that extends into the vagina). The vagina is automatically shortened if the cervix is removed, although if a surgical technique called "Worrelling" is used, most of its length can be preserved. If the surgeon doesn't use the proper technique to dissect the cervix from the vagina, scarring can also occur. Vaginal tissue can stretch, but scar tissue cannot. Generally, if a woman facing hysterectomy insists on keeping her cervix, she can keep the length of her vagina intact.

There are other good reasons for retaining the cervix. It helps support the pelvic floor structures; for example, it will help prevent the bladder from prolapsing, or becoming displaced and/or distended. It can act as a barrier for infection and provides some vaginal lubrication. If a woman retains her cervix, her vaginal integrity is more likely to remain stable. Given the significant role that the cervix plays in a woman's general and sexual well-being, it is unfortunate that women contemplating hysterectomy are rarely informed of the complications that can ensue if it is removed.

In its 1999 pamphlet on *Understanding Hysterectomy*, the American College of Obstetricians and Gynecologists (ACOG) states clearly that if the hysterectomy procedure requires vaginal shortening, deep thrusting with intercourse may become painful. It makes the following two recommendations: 1) *Being on top during sex or* 2) *bringing your legs closer together may help.* Any woman will tell you that intercourse wouldn't be pleasurable, if at all possible, if she had to keep her legs closer together, and women living with the condition of a shortened vagina will tell you that attempting the "on top" position would be excruciatingly painful. That's why it is so important to get all the facts on post-hysterectomy sexuality before you get to the operating room.

Complications from perforations and shortened vaginas are discussed in no fewer than five of the stories featured in this book (including my own). Contrary to popular belief, a woman's sex life may not improve after her hysterectomy. Women and their lovers must seriously consider a potential reduction in the quality of sexual function as a major side effect of hysterectomy.

Weight Gain

According to Elizabeth Plourde, author of *Hysterectomy and Ovary Removal: What ALL Women Need to KNOW*, 14 to 28 percent of hysterectomized women report problems of either weight gain or weight loss. Unfortunately, many doctors believe that weight gain following hysterectomy has psychological causes. New research confirms that, when unopposed by progesterone or testosterone, estrogen in the form of hormone replacement therapy does cause weight gain in many hysterectomized women.

I gained more than forty pounds in the years following my hysterectomy. No doctor had ever told me about the risk of weight gain or asked me whether I wanted to live the rest of my life with excessive poundage around my middle. The resulting stares and comments about my weight have had a truly detrimental effect on my self-esteem.

If a woman gains weight after her hysterectomy, it is important for her to remember that her problem is very likely directly linked to the disruption of her hormonal balance. Hysterectomized and oophorectomized women who would like to lose post-surgical weight should seek the help of a doctor who recognizes this alteration in their biochemistry.

Generalized Fatigue and Insomnia

Because of generalized fatigue, I find it increasingly difficult to work a full day without rest. I experience repeated "shutdown" periods when it feels as though a magnet is pulling away the little energy I have. Countless women I have talked to report the same energy deficit. Fatigue may be the result of sleep interrupted by night sweats and depression.

But even when they get extra, uninterrupted sleep at night, some women always feel exhausted.

Hormone Replacement Therapy (HRT)

A woman's ovaries produce estrogen, progesterone, and testosterone; they are her main source of hormones. When the ovaries, which are equivalent to a man's testes, are removed, women cease to produce hormones. They have, in effect, been surgically castrated.

While the uterus does not produce any hormones, it shares a blood supply with the ovaries and cervix, and is intricately involved with the ovaries in hormonal health. According to Montreal-based compounding pharmacist Mel Alter, if the blood supply going to the ovaries is damaged at hysterectomy, women who retained those organs may lose ovarian function within two or three years.

Without a uterus and/or ovaries, most women will go into menopause earlier than they would have if surgery had been avoided. As I have discussed above, the symptoms of surgical menopause are many, can range from mild to quite severe, and are often more pronounced in women who are surgically castrated than in those who lose ovarian function gradually, through natural menopause.

Traditionally, hysterectomized and oophorectomized women have been prescribed estrogen replacement therapy (ERT) to help control the symptoms of surgical menopause. The most common therapy is a drug called Premarin, which is made from the urine of pregnant mares. This is the drug I was prescribed following my hysterectomy. Estradiol, CES, and Ogen are other estrogen supplements, which are often used in combination with progesterone or progestin if the woman has retained her uterus.

While ERT works well for some women, it is not a cure-all; many women do not respond, or respond well, to these drugs, and can develop a range of side effects. The possible unwanted effects of conventional estrogen replacement are usually the symptoms of excess estrogen; they can include breast tenderness, headaches, leg cramps, gallstones, worsening of uterine fibroids and endometriosis, vaginal bleeding, high blood pressure, blood clots, nausea and vomiting, fluid retention, impaired glucose tolerance, and increased risk of sex-organ cancers. Dr. Cutler writes,

> If you take HRT incorrectly, side effects are your signal that the dosage needs to be changed. Since your body is different from anyone else's, the amount of hormone that you need to maximize your hormonal balance will be unique to you. Once you understand how hormones influence your body, you will become sensitive to your own dosage options.[10]

Of greater concern, is the fact that we now have strong evidence that long term use of HRT is not safe. It can lead to an increased risk of breast cancer, heart disease, stroke and blood clots. This information was released in July 2002, by the U.S. National Heart, Lung and Blood Institution, after it abruptly halted its most significant study to date into the effects of hormone replacement therapy.

Long term use of HRT is not an option for women whose ovaries are surgically removed. And of course now that our suspicions about HRT have been confirmed, the decision to retain or remove non-cancerous ovaries should be weighed very carefully.

Human estrogen, explains Mel Alter, consists naturally of three estrogens in varying proportions: estriol (60 to 80 percent), estradiol (10 to 20 percent), and estrone (10 to 20 percent). Estrogens derived from animal sources, such as Premarin, and estrogen supplements that use only one form of estrogen aren't natural and don't accurately mimic a woman's pre-surgery hormonal production. Many estrogen supplements, he says, are too strong for many women.

Natural hormone replacement therapy (NHRT) may be one solution

---

10 Cutler, Winnifred B. *Hysterectomy Before and After: A Comprehensive Guide to Preventing, Preparing for, and Maximizing Health After Hysterectomy.* (New York: HarperCollins, 1989), 129.

for women who want to avoid traditional E/HRT or who have not responded well to traditional treatments. Natural hormone therapy means that the chemical makeup of the replacement hormone is exactly the same as that produced by the human body. It combines all three estrogens that the ovaries generate naturally in what is known as the "tri-est" formula: usually 80 percent estriol, 10 percent estradiol, and 10 percent estrone.

In NHRT, says Mr. Alter, estrogen is always opposed with natural micronized progesterone, which has a calming effect on the brain, promotes new bone growth, and protects breast tissue from excessive stimulation by estrogen. We have receptors for progesterone not only in the uterus, but also in the bones, breast tissue, brain, and elsewhere; clearly it is necessary for health beyond its function in the uterus.

Progestins (such as MPA and Provera), which are synthetic versions of progesterone often found in HRT, can also cause many side effects, including headaches, depression, weight gain and bloating, moodiness, low libido, heart disease, and acne. As well, progestins do not protect women against coronary vasoconstriction as does natural progesterone, nor do they have progesterone's beneficial effect on the bones. Synthetic progestins can also inhibit the beneficial effects of estrogen therapy on HDL, or "good" cholesterol. Natural micronized progesterone has a much lower negative effect on HDL-C than does MPA (Medroxi Progesterone Acetate) as shown in the Post-menopausal Estrogen/ Progestin Interventions (PEPI) study conducted by the Women's Health Initiative (WHI) and funded by the U.S. National Institutes of Health, released on February 6, 1996.

Natural hormone replacement therapy can also include, when needed, testosterone and/or the hormone DHEA in doses appropriate for the individual woman. Most hysterectomized women, explains Mr. Alter, need testosterone, which cannot be supplied through conventional HRT. They must get it either in monthly injections, which are inconvenient, or through NHRT.

Compounding pharmacists such as Mel Alter can compound, or mix together, natural, bio-identical hormones derived from plants. By compounding, the practitioner can create a customized medication in the form that suits the patient best: topical cream, sustained release capsules, sublingual drops, or troches. In consultation with a woman and her physician, a compounding pharmacist can prepare a made-to-measure hormonal mixture that best suits her needs and wishes. European physicians have prescribed compounded hormones for more than fifty years.

Unfortunately, it can be difficult to get a doctor to prescribe NHRT. Most doctors are not well informed about natural hormones, says Mr. Alter. Drug companies, he points out, will not promote or do studies on products that cannot be patented, and these include natural hormones. As well, compounded medications do not have drug identification numbers (DINs) and are not included in the Compendium of Pharmaceutical Specialties (CPS), because no pharmaceutical companies produce natural hormones. Since the CPS is the source doctors use for information on available drugs, and since they are hesitant to prescribe medications about which they are not fully informed or that do not have DIN numbers, they tend not to prescribe compounded hormones. They fear pressure from their medical boards or problems with insurance. "They do not understand that these hormones are real hormones and real medicine," says Mr. Alter.[11]

It is not an easy task to find a medical specialist willing to monitor a hysterectomized woman's progress on this form of therapy, but it is possible. It took me a one-year search to finally find a compounding pharmacist in Canada. Most compounding pharmacists can direct women to physicians who are knowledgeable and willing to prescribe NHRT. To find one in your area, contact the International Academy of Compounding Pharmacists (IACP) at 1-800-927-4227, or Professional Compounding Centers of America at 1-800-331-2498. In Canada, contact Wiler-PCCA at 1-800-668-9453.

---

11 Mel Alter, BSc, Phm, LPh, FACA, Montréal, QC, Canada. Interview with Susan Goldberg, November 2001.

Finding the right specialist to prescribe the proper form and dosage of hormonal replacement therapy can involve a long journey. However, for women who suffer greatly from the adverse effects of surgical menopause, it is a vitally important path that can help lead them back towards the quality of life they enjoyed before surgery.

"Many women are not fully informed about their bodies and the options they have," says Mel Alter. "They should read and inform themselves *before* surgery. If doctors used natural progesterone at the right time, whether for PMS, at the first sign of perimenopause or fibroids, for excessive bleeding or endometriosis, I believe that most hysterectomies could be avoided."[12]

Informed Consent

Without a thorough understanding of all the risks and benefits associated with hysterectomy, a woman cannot give her informed consent to the operation. Women must ask their doctors about the risk factors before surgery, and doctors must provide women with full and complete answers, including information on alternative courses of treatment. If your doctor is unwilling to discuss the risks of hysterectomy, oophorectomy, or any other surgery recommended for you, seek a second medical opinion.

The decision whether to undergo hysterectomy properly rests with the woman whose bodily integrity is at stake, says Dr. Cutler.

> [She] will be guided by her own knowledge and judgment, by the counsel she requests, by those who live with her and love her, and by a compassionate physician, whose diagnosis should always be reinforced by a second opinion from another doctor who has no stake in the first opinion. . . . Physicians must learn to respect both the intelligence and the dignity of their patients. Doctors must lead patients

---

12 Mel Alter, BSc, Phm, LPh, FACA, Montréal, QC, Canada. Interview with Susan Goldberg, November 2001.

to information, and work with them, serving in the role of professional consultant. Only then can the patient exert a free and truly informed choice.[13]

At the end of this book you will find a list of questions that might be helpful to women considering a hysterectomy. I know that if I had to do it all over again, I would ask my gynecologist those questions again and again until I had a clear understanding of all the consequences that can arise from this surgery. Had I known what I know now, I might have made very different choices.

Your personal health care is an important responsibility. Ask your questions, and insist on answers before you sign a consent form for any type of surgery. If you aren't happy with the answers you receive, or if the risks seem too great, you may want to seek a second opinion or pursue alternative therapies. Your present and future health and well-being are at stake.

The views expressed in this book are those of the individual contributors, and may be contrary to the opinions of some medical professionals. The primary intent of this work is to inform, in the hope that women facing hysterectomy will be encouraged to research this procedure and its potential consequences. The underlying objective is that awareness about our difficulties will lead to further research into treatments to help women better cope with the negative outcomes of hysterectomy.

---

13 Cutler, Winnifred B. *Hysterectomy Before and After: A Comprehensive Guide to Preventing, Preparing for, and Maximizing Health After Hysterectomy.* (New York: HarperCollins, 1989), 11.

PART II

Our Stories

Introduction

❦

MARY ANNE WYATT OF MASSACHUSETTS

"Wei was to discover that he had joined a group of peculiar people who were neither men nor women. With his natural male forces abated, the fundamental process of biological change occurred in his body cells, evidenced in changed functions and in appearance. There was an apparent loss of height and beard, his nose became broader, and his ear lobes thicker. Decreasing hormone levels caused a loss of elasticity: his skin wrinkled, his joints stiffened, and his muscle strength gradually weakened. . . . Although not readily visible to him, perhaps the most important changes occurred in the lungs and the cardiovascular systems. These led to a decrease in his body's ability to gather oxygen from the air, and a decreased ability to pump adequate blood with its essential components to all parts of his body. He soon became soft and fat."[14]

— *ACCOUNT OF A PALACE EUNUCH OF THE MING DYNASTY (LATE SIXTEENTH CENTURY)*

---

14 Tsai, Shih-shan Henry. *The Eunuchs in the Ming Dynasty.* (New York: State University of New York Press, 1996), 4.

Writing about hysterectomy was not easy for any of the contributors to this book, including me. It is hard to articulate so much hidden pain. These heart-wrenching stories come from the souls of women who were catapulted via surgery into a world we had not expected and about which no one had warned us. Through sharing our stories with others, we have come to recognize that many of our symptoms are not unique, but systemic, even predictable, and that we are not alone. We share our stories here in the hope that those who are considering hysterectomy and women who have been hysterectomized will find within these pages information, strength, resources, and a community of empathetic women.

How We Feel

We are alive, but in different selves. Many of us feel like outcasts from our previous lives. Too many of us grieve for loss of spirit, vitality, identity, the birthright of innate femininity, and the pure joys of sexual awareness. Most of us had never questioned the inherent gift of sexual desire until it was excised surgically from our bodies. Now our sex lives are different: some of us had doctors who surgically shortened our vaginas during surgery, making penetrative sex difficult or painful. Some of us experience dryness and pain, or a simple lack of interest in sex. Many of us have experienced the hurt of fractured romantic relationships.

The world has lost much of its former lustre and excitement. Our senses and emotions are deadened — we feel flat when we view a lovely work of art or hear a romantic Rachmaninoff symphony. Some of us have lost maternal feeling towards our children, our eagerness to be touched and hugged, and even the lusty enjoyment of good perfume.

Many of us have gained weight. We hate being fat, losing our hair, aging rapidly. Our clothes don't fit. We compare ourselves to movie heroines in their beautiful clothes. Old romantic songs surround and haunt us. It becomes harder to care.

For many, sadness is never far away. Depression can be a major consequence of our surgeries. For some, it becomes difficult to separate depression from despair. We become reclusive. We tend to hide, to disappear from friends and acquaintances. Our bodies are seeking to re-establish biochemical equilibrium from a discordant cacophony of hormones. We feel disconnected and un-whole, floundering in an ocean of hormone choices and supplements, with no reliable, consistent solutions. Meanwhile, our bodies continue to cycle and change.

We experience incapacitating hot flashes and drenching night sweats. We lose brushfuls of hair. Our skin dries out. We suffer from debilitating headaches, bone and muscle pain, fatigue, and insomnia. Hysterectomy has compromised our immune systems, so we suffer more allergies and are sick more often. Our uteruses secreted an irreplaceable hormone that protected our hearts. Without our natural ovarian hormones, we are at higher risk of developing arthritis, osteoporosis, and fibromyalgia.

Many of us have suffered injuries to the urinary tract, the bowel, and pelvic nerves and structures. Surgeons have perforated our tissues. Bladder and ureter injuries are a known risk of hysterectomy, as is some degree of incontinence, the result of damaged or weakened pelvic-floor muscles and nerves. Many of us live with "broken glass" in our bladders. We never imagined we would have to wear Depends to prevent wetting ourselves while chasing our toddlers or attending formal dinner parties.

We have been referred to psychologists and psychiatrists for what are obviously physical injuries, have been told that it's "all in our heads," and have had our pain greeted with guilt-driven anger or abuse from doctors. Many of us have been told that our new injuries were pre-existing conditions, or have been given diagnoses that do not fit. Our treatments have been delayed, and some of us have been abandoned by the very "health care" system that injured us.

Many of us have left much loved and needed productive careers and are now struggling to work and survive financially on reduced incomes — while our medical bills mount. Others of us have been forced to put aside plans for further education. Many of us were still raising our families at the time of our surgery, and took our healthy future for granted.

We have discovered gross violations of medical ethics. Residents bartered for our bodies even before we were anesthetized. Some women have found out that surgical equipment salesmen or other non-skilled personnel were allowed to operate on them, without their knowledge or consent. Others have discovered that the doctors who performed their surgery were not surgeons or gynecologists but general practitioners, or worse, representatives of pharmaceutical companies, without adequate surgical training. Medical records have been altered or omitted from our files.

Many of us feel justifiable anger and rage. It is impossible to be "nice" in the face of injustice. We have wrongly blamed ourselves and have been made to feel stupid. We are intelligent women who believed what we were told by authority figures we trusted.

What We Were — and Weren't — Told

Historically, our biology has been a prisoner of sexual oppression. Menstruation and pregnancy were treated as diseases, childbirth required surgical intervention, and menopause was a death. The word "hysteria" comes from the Greek word for uterus, and in the nineteenth century that organ, believed to be the source of women's "hysterical" nature, was cause for psychoanalytic treatment or surgical excision.

How far have we really come today? Medicine continues to describe normal hormonal fluctuations such as premenstrual syndrome as psychiatric disorders, or to treat them with surgery. Society condones epidemic numbers of hysterectomies, and allows doctors to routinely remove healthy ovaries for absolutely no medical reason.

In general, we did not have life-threatening problems. We were robbed of appropriate medical options for addressing our problems. Many of us gave in to surgery reluctantly, out of fear and because of persuasion by doctors in a paternalistic medical system. Others agreed to surgery readily; we believed our surgeons when they told us that hysterectomy was a routine procedure with minimal consequences. We trusted our doctors, male and female, as individuals and caretakers. But they have been too easily swayed by the market forces of drug companies or by departments of surgery eager to provide training opportunities for residents — at too high a cost.

Most of us were told that losing our uterus or our ovaries would not affect us sexually. We were sold the myth that simple hormone replacement — some combination of usually synthetic versions of estrogen, progesterone, and testosterone — could easily replace the complex functions of our lost organs. Others of us were told that we would simply experience menopause.

As a group, we have been casually relegated to the trash bin of "surgical menopause," a convenient, albeit inaccurate, phrase. Few of us, however, were prepared for the shock of this process. Our menopausal realities hardly match those of the smiling, grey-haired women in the magazine ads! At any age, there is nothing natural about surgical cutoff of the pathways between our genitals and our brain. We were not told that menopause is a gradual process that can take over ten years to complete, or that it should be characterized not by failure of our sexual organs, but rather as a miraculous change in their function, on a continuum.

Many of us were told that hysterectomy and oophorectomy would prevent cancer. Why should we care more about the phantom risk of cancer than about losing our energy, looks, youth, and sexual happiness? Chemical castration is considered cruel and unusual punishment for male sex offenders, yet doctors do not consider that healthy women might treasure their genitals and their sexual well-being. When there is no proven pathology and where other good alternatives exist, hysterectomy is wholesale sexual mutilation.

Hope and Change

There is hope, because we are finally coming to grips with the truth. Without accurate information, women cannot give informed consent to the physical and emotional consequences of hysterectomy. We need laws that mandate informed consent for this life-altering surgery. We need consent forms that detail both the short- and long-term implications, that we can take home for careful consideration. We should have the option of videos of our pelvic surgeries to review later with our doctors. It may be time to suggest that doctors must prove pathology before proceeding with any surgery.

We will seek medical advice only from doctors who treat us with dignity and respect. We want full information in order to make our own choices, and to wrest back control over the fate of our sex organs. When we do choose surgery, we want safe operations by expert, qualified surgeons who will take the time to remove only diseased tissue and only when its removal is necessary for continuance of life. Anything less is disrespectful.

Some of us have had repair work done by qualified surgeons, and some varying degrees of improvement have been attained with the help of radiologists, endocrinologists, and practitioners of integrative medicine. Endocrinologists, who specialize in endocrine dysfunction and hormone balance, can steer us to options other than hysterectomy. Complete endocrine profiles can help determine hormone imbalances before and after hysterectomy, and home testing kits are now available to test for hormone levels by using urine or saliva. Good support networks are being formed to help us discover these options.

New drug delivery systems make it possible to prescribe and compound a variety of natural hormones, personalized for individual women. Many of us have found that natural hormones (recognized as biochemically similar to those that our own bodies once generated) work better, and with fewer side effects, than synthetic drugs. Women need the option of natural hormone replacement therapy and comprehensive information on the subject. Fortunately, they have begun to receive it.

We are learning the importance not only of estrogen and progesterone, but also of the action and interaction of hormones such as
DHEA, testosterone, prolactin, melatonin, and growth hormone, of
human pheromones, the peptides oxytocin and vasopressin, and other
ingredients that work in synchronicity in the chemical soup that is our
bodies. Together, these ingredients can have anti-aging effects and promote sexual well-being.

Women with pelvic-floor injuries may be able to get some relief from
qualified physical therapists who can assess the origins of nerve, muscle,
and soft-tissue pain. New radiology techniques such as magnetic resonance neurography (MRN) can visualize injured nerves. Rehabilitation
with trigger-point therapy and deep tissue mobilization can help alleviate pain, prevent incontinence, and restore blood supply to areas of
the pelvis traumatized by surgery. These treatments should be considered as soon as possible after surgery. Women have succumbed to losing
all of their pelvic organs, including their bladders, before discovering
that the pain had been caused all along by constriction of muscles surrounding those organs.

The possibilities of ovarian transplant instead of oophorectomy,
nerve-sparing surgery, and careful imaging of the uterine and ovarian
blood supply prior to hysterectomy could spare women from the consequences of hysterectomy that so many of us describe in this book.

We are still responsible for ensuring that the range of treatment
options — before and after hysterectomy — continues to expand. We
must demand that women no longer be used as practice subjects for
medical school residents. We must demand that surgeons be held
accountable for what they do to us. We must insist on a follow-up
system for post-hysterectomy patients that can lead them to valid sources
of help. The millions of women who have had hysterectomies form an
enormous constituency that warrants long-term epidemiological study.

Finally, we must continue to empower ourselves with information.
Only when we are aware of all the possible consequences and alternatives to hysterectomy can we make truly informed choices. For all this,

we need the support of our loved ones, our friends, and our families, more than they can know.

About Mary Anne Wyatt

Mary Anne Wyatt's career has embraced both a passion for scientific research and a deep and abiding interest in the betterment of her community. In addition to researching molecular biology for six years at the Massachusetts Institute of Technology, Mary Anne has worked extensively in the private sector as a chemist in the tangential fields of physical and inorganic chemistry and electrochemistry.

Mary Anne has maintained an ongoing commitment to a wide range of humanitarian causes. She has been a board member and president of several non-profit organizations, including the Florence Crittenton League for women with unplanned pregnancies, the Orenda Wildlife Trust and other conservation societies, and the New England Banjo Society. In 1989 Mary Anne was awarded the Humanitarian of the Year distinction by the Animal Protection Institute of America.

Lise:

My Own Story

❧

I remember several of my Grade 7 and 8 classmates bragging about their exciting experiences as they officially entered the world of womanhood. My own entrance into that world, however, was not a happy event. From the time I started menstruating at the age of twelve, I had problems with pelvic pain, numbness in my legs, abdominal swelling, and migraines. Perhaps some of my classmates were exaggerating about their wonderful transformations and felt as bad as I did. In any case, it would be interesting to meet and talk with some of them today to find out if any of their menstrual histories were as eventful as mine over the years.

I almost always spent the first couple of days of my period in bed, with my legs raised to curb the excessive flow of blood. I continued to suffer greatly from painful menses until my family physician put me on the birth control pill at the age of fifteen. Finally, I had relief from that nightmarish monthly experience. But if I went off the contraceptives, all my problems came back with a vengeance.

Many older women told me that my painful menses would be a thing of the past once I had given birth. Not so in my case. In fact, the pain I experienced at menstruation became even more severe in my late twenties, even though I had been through two pregnancies — pregnancies that were considered high risk, and during which I suffered from toxemia and many other ailments.

At the time, I was trapped in a difficult first marriage, which didn't help matters any. I wasn't allowed to be sick, nor was I allowed to complain. I kept my menstrual difficulties to myself, and went back on the pill after each pregnancy. It continued to be effective in alleviating my pain and controlling the excessive blood flow.

At the age of thirty-two, I came across some literature on the increased risk of blood clots in women who continued to take the pill into their thirties. This new knowledge prompted me to stop taking the drug, but the excruciating pain that came with my next period made me wish I had never found the article. I went back to missing a couple of days of work each month, a situation I found both difficult and embarrassing to explain to my superiors and colleagues.

I was single again at that point, and trying to rebuild a new life for my boys and myself. Part of that new life included dating and, naturally, sex. Now that I was off the pill, I needed a new form of birth control. I sought the advice of a gynecologist, who recommended a tubal ligation. Given my history of high-risk pregnancies and my two Caesarean sections, I couldn't see myself having another baby. The gynecologist agreed that another pregnancy would not be a wise choice for me, so I had my tubes tied in the spring of 1984.

I had hoped that the tubal ligation might give me some relief from the pain I experienced each month, although I don't think there is any medical reason why it should have. Of course, it did not. Later I read research reports showing that tubal sterilization often results in further menstrual problems, as well as hormonal imbalance, which is exactly what started happening to me. I have since come across studies suggesting that tubal ligation can damage blood vessels, thus compromising ovarian function and possibly resulting in the early onset of menopause.

Other risks associated with the procedure include the accidental perforation of organs, pelvic inflammatory disease (PID), premenstrual syndrome (PMS), and painful and heavier menses.

I began experiencing what I believed to be PMS symptoms before, during, and after my period. Often my symptoms were worst the week *after* my period. Later I read that this week is normally the best time of the month for women with premenstrual syndrome; the pattern of my cycle suggested that my problems were not all related to PMS.[15] My symptoms were more or less constant, and they became more pronounced throughout my early and mid-thirties. My family will readily attest that living with me then was not unlike witnessing a weekly Jekyll-and-Hyde transformation. I would feel thunder rumbling from within before I lost all control over my emotions, venting my rage and moods on whomever was nearest. Then I would sink into a deep depression because I knew that I had hurt those around me. I couldn't understand why I overreacted to every little crisis.

High stress levels can affect hormonal balance, and several other factors had a role in my overall emotional and physical well-being at the time. I was getting over the end of my first marriage and recent divorce, for instance. My elder son suffered from attention deficit disorder (ADD), while my youngest had started to stutter at the age of three. My sons' teachers had considerable difficulty coping with their disorders, often resulting in unpleasant experiences for them at school, and for me as well.

As a single mother of two, staying at home was not an option. I provided for my children through contract communications work. Those short-term jobs were demanding, stressful positions that made it more difficult for me to cope with the havoc of my personal life. As I networked and looked for job opportunities, my self-esteem took a beating from the constant rejections. I felt incredibly overwhelmed and depressed at times. Perhaps it isn't surprising that my symptoms weren't necessarily all PMS-related.

---

15 West, Stanley, with Paula Dranov. *The Hysterectomy Hoax*. (New Jersey, Next Decade, Inc., 2002), 158.

It Had to Stop

By the mid-1980s, there were only three or four days in a month when it was safe for me to go out or to be around people. My menstrual flow was continuous and abundant. I was irritable and I experienced abrupt mood swings, especially in times of high stress. My legs were weak and I had constant pain in my lower back. I gained eight or ten pounds a month from bloating before and during my period, and the challenge of losing the weight before the next period of bloat left me depressed and feeling inadequate and worthless.

I was feeling that my health difficulties made it almost impossible for anyone to love me. Meeting Paul, therefore, made me feel truly fortunate. I needed acceptance and understanding in a way that I had assumed most men would find difficult to provide. As I look back on the many trying situations that characterized the early years of our relationship, I wonder to this day why Paul asked me to marry him in 1988. These days, I try not to question his love for me; above all else, it's what keeps me going. He's still my reason for getting up in the morning, even though there are many days when I don't have the will to do anything or go anywhere.

In the meantime, my escalating menstrual problems had to stop. In my search for a solution, I agreed to see my parents' family physician. According to them, she was a young doctor who really seemed to care about her patients. I know now that I would have been better off finding a good physician on my own, but I hadn't heard of shopping around for a qualified specialist.

After I discussed my painful menses with her during my first visit, the doctor claimed that I might have endometriosis. She recommended a total abdominal hysterectomy and bilateral salpingo-oophorectomy (TAHBSO) — in other words, the surgical removal of my uterus, cervix, Fallopian tubes, and ovaries — and referred me to a gynecological surgeon.

My doctor explained to me that a hysterectomy would put an end to all my pain at menstruation. So determined was she to sell me on the idea of a hysterectomy that she told me I could avoid all risks of uterine, ovarian, and cervical cancer. I bought this line of thinking, but, if I could turn back the clock, I would now reply that it simply doesn't make sense to remove essential body parts — just in case they might become cancerous in the future!

Why the Rush?

The doctor asked to see me with my husband within the next couple of weeks in order to discuss the procedure with both of us. Though this would have been an excellent opportunity for her to discuss the likelihood of depression and loss of libido after a hysterectomy, she did not. She said that I would be entering into the wonderful world of menopause and added that hormone replacement therapy (HRT) would help me live happily ever after — no more painful menstruation and no more endometriosis.

One of my main concerns about the hysterectomy was the risk of gaining weight. All the women that my mother knew who had had hysterectomies had become obese. But the three specialists involved in my case (the family physician, the gynecologist, and the chief of gynecological surgery, whom I met just once before my surgery) indicated that there was *absolutely no risk* of weight gain after the surgery. "If you don't put it in your mouth, you won't gain," said the gynecologist. Both he and the family physician told me that weight gain caused by a hysterectomy was nothing but an old wives' tale.

During my visits to the gynecologist's office, I couldn't help but notice his hyperactivity. He was almost always hours behind schedule, his waiting room was usually full, and he would literally run from one patient room to the next. Consequently, I didn't feel comfortable trying to discuss all my concerns carefully with him. This alone should have given me sufficient reason to run in the other direction.

To help me decide whether or not to proceed with a hysterectomy, the gynecologist proposed the Zoladex treatment, whereby I would receive monthly abdominal injections that would result in the cessation of my menstrual flow and, inevitably, the onset of severe menopausal symptoms. This was in 1991. Zoladex was initially approved in Canada and the United States for the treatment of prostate cancer in 1989. In 1993, it was approved in Canada for the treatment of endometriosis; other approvals have followed since for further treatments for endometriosis and for advanced breast cancer in pre- and perimenopausal women.

Although I understood that I was to undergo a hysterectomy for pelvic pain, or endometriosis, the gynecologist now claims that I was hysterectomized for mood swings related to PMS. Yet he was proposing to treat me with a drug to manage endometriosis — two years before its approval for that use in Canada. He never obtained my consent to take part in what now appears to have been a clinical trial for an as-yet-unapproved drug. And he never performed an exploratory laparoscopy to determine if I really had the disease before going ahead with its treatment.

Zoladex's product monograph lists the following side effects: hot flushes, mood swings, decreased libido, sweating, insomnia, depression, nervousness, pelvic pain, and weight gain, among many others. I find it interesting that the gynecologist would opt to treat me with a drug whose potential side effects were identical to some of the symptoms from which I was seeking relief. Still, I took the Zoladex. The results were nearly unbearable. Heat flooded from my lower abdomen to the top of my head every five or six minutes, making it impossible for me to leave the house for a period of three months. I didn't have air conditioning at home, so I spent most of my days standing with my head in the freezer compartment of our fridge. The night sweats were just as severe.

When I asked the gynecologist if I would have to endure that level of discomfort after the hysterectomy, he said that I would not. I would be on estrogen replacement therapy, he told me, which would completely free me of those symptoms. I wondered, then, why he had prescribed the discomforts of Zoladex treatment in the first place, if it wouldn't give me an accurate picture of post-hysterectomy life.

I was stuck between a rock and a hard place — I didn't want to go back to my painful and prolonged menses, and I wanted the flushing and mild anxiety attacks that came with the Zoladex treatments to stop at any cost. I agreed to undergo surgery. I now feel that the circumstances under which I made that decision were highly unusual, and strained at best. I certainly did not get all the facts about this life-changing operation.

The gynecologist did not provide any warnings about the effects of surgical menopause. I asked him why I couldn't hang on to my ovaries. After all, I thought, my uterus was the only organ affected by the endometriosis. He didn't explain that removal of my ovaries would double my risk of osteoporosis and extinguish my sexual desire. Nor did he warn me against the severe side effects of ERT. He simply replied that removing my ovaries was the only option that would get rid of my PMS symptoms at the same time.

I have not come across any medical literature or other information since that supports this view in any regard. However, I have read a great deal of material that explains why PMS is *not* a justifiable reason for hysterectomy or oophorectomy. In dismissing my concerns and in neglecting to investigate whether any of my symptoms could be linked to PMS, the gynecologist ignored the fact that the ovaries produce testosterone and progesterone, both hormones that strongly influence a woman's sexual desire and energy.

It is interesting to note how one doctor's view differs from that of another. In 1999, for example, a different gynecologist told me that if a woman suffers from depression and PMS before a hysterectomy, she will continue to suffer from those same symptoms afterwards. If I had come to him in 1991, he said, he would have told me exactly that. Since I continue to suffer from depression and PMS-like symptoms, I have no doubt that this specialist was right. My hysterectomy seemed only to compound the problem. More importantly, given my history of depression, I most certainly was not a good candidate for the operation.

Post-hysterectomy Blues

My recovery in the hospital went well. The gynecologist who performed the surgery prescribed a daily dose of three milligrams of Premarin before I went home from the hospital. The dose prescribed was obviously too high for me, because my breasts started aching almost immediately. The swelling and tenderness in my breasts (a condition called mastalgia) was so painful that I had to cross my arms in front of my chest to go up or down a flight of stairs. When I reported this symptom during my post-op visit with the gynecologist, he told me to take my problems back to my family physician. What a great bedside manner!

I live with the discomfort of mastalgia to this day. It seems to be a side effect of every different form of estrogen I have tried to date, regardless of the dose. "Like any medical therapy," writes Dr. Judith Reichman in *I'm Too Young to Get Old*, "estrogen can cause adverse effects, especially if it is improperly prescribed or not sufficiently monitored. . . . If ERT could help [women] achieve good hearts, healthy bones, well-functioning bladders, enjoyable sex, and wrinkle-free skin without side effects or risks, we would not be struggling with our individual hormone decisions."[16] There are many forms of estrogen on the market, notes Dr. Reichman, and women who develop unpleasant symptoms from one form are well advised to try another.[17] Unfortunately, my doctor did not give me that option. And, at that time, I didn't know that other types of estrogen were available.

To relieve the discomfort of mastalgia, I had breast reduction surgery in March 1994, which provided some relief for a couple of years. However, given my hypersensitivity to ERT, the symptoms have returned in recent years, and my discomfort is much greater. I am likely due for a second breast reduction, once more undergoing the physical risks, stresses, and trauma of surgery.

---

16 Reichman, Judith. *I'm Too Young to Get Old: Health Care for Women After Forty*. (New York: Random House, 1996), 139.
17 Reichman, 156.

Just four months after my hysterectomy, I reported to my family physician that sexual intercourse was difficult and painful. She promptly provided me with a few tips on foreplay. Although I felt like telling her that I didn't need a how-to lesson, I sat through her Sex 101 crash course, not saying much. Instead, I had a highly charged conversation with myself in the car on the way home, berating myself for not telling her how insulting her advice had been. In retrospect, her response wasn't that surprising; most of the doctors I have seen associate sexual dysfunction with a psychological disorder. I knew that my problem was physical, and yet I hadn't insisted on a physical examination.

Noticing the Changes

One year later and nineteen pounds heavier, I found myself losing all interest in sex. When I again raised the subject with my doctor, she dismissed my concerns once more. Painful intercourse was not the only problem I had; my libido was all but extinguished. Somehow I knew that my family physician couldn't provide any solutions. I don't think she knew enough about surgical menopause to connect loss of libido with the removal of my ovaries, and especially not with the ERT. According to her, a daily dose of estrogen was the solution to all my problems. It didn't seem to matter to her that my hypersensitivity to Premarin would cause further weight gain, which would in turn result in lower self-esteem and deeper depression.

When I went for a routine mammogram in 1993, it showed a small lesion in my left breast, which was surgically removed in November. This frightened me enormously. I knew that the ERT had more than likely caused the lesion, which had appeared just two years after I started my daily doses of Premarin. I thought that I had no choice but to keep on taking this drug for the rest of my life, and this worried me immensely. I worried about the risk of breast cancer every time I popped a Premarin tablet in my mouth or rubbed my belly with the EstroGel (another estrogen supplement) that I was using in early 1999.

I continued with the ERT because without it, the severity of the flushes and the deep depression I would experience tended to provoke thoughts of suicide.

In spite of sensible eating, my weight continued to climb, making me all the more depressed. My family physician explained that I belonged to the "very small group of women" who *do* experience negative side effects from ERT. She told me that she had not been overly concerned that I would gain weight or experience any other symptoms while taking Premarin. According to her, very few women have adverse side effects from this drug. Sadly, many doctors still hold this view today. Yet about a quarter of all women on ERT report gaining weight, especially in the abdominal area. Now that more women are speaking out about menopausal symptoms, we may find out that the percentage is actually higher. As well, women whose ovaries are surgically removed reportedly suffer far more serious menopausal symptoms than women who lose ovarian function gradually through natural menopause.[18]

My family physician also told me that Premarin is practically the same as the birth control pill. Because I was prone to gaining weight on the pill, said the doctor, I should have guessed that I would gain weight on ERT. Unfortunately, I didn't know about the similarities between these drug treatments. My doctor should have given me that information before she talked me into the hysterectomy.

I sought treatment for my depression in 1994, and was prescribed Prozac. I found out later that Prozac also causes weight gain in many people who take it, and can lead to obesity in others. I also discovered that antidepressants such as Prozac, Zoloft, and Paxil can cause loss of libido. It's ironic. I sought psychiatric treatment for depression brought on by surgical removal of my ovaries and exacerbated by the resulting weight gain and loss of libido. I was then prescribed a drug with the side

---

18 Curtis, A.H., M.D., and J.W. Huffman, M.D.. *A Textbook of Gynecology*, (Philadelphia: W.B. Saunders Company HB, 1950), 103: "The castration menopause is generally stated to be the same as the natural menopause. In our experience, it differs in that it varies much more in its intensity. The vigor of some castrated patients appears to help them to withstand the menopause without discomfort. In other cases, the reaction is rather violent and requires large doses of estrogen for the control of symptoms."

effects of weight gain and loss of libido, effectively maintaining the status quo!

Persistent Symptoms

In spite of dieting and exercising, I gained an additional twenty pounds during the second and third years after my hysterectomy. Since I was taking both Premarin and Prozac at the time, it's difficult to know which caused the weight gain. Whatever the cause, I was getting heavier, and felt less desirable than ever. Feeling very alone, I decided to seek the help of another doctor. Between 1993 and 1995, I visited at least four physicians, and each felt that all I needed was a good psychiatrist.

Meanwhile, the aftereffects of my hysterectomy were becoming more significant, though I had not yet connected most of them with my 1991 surgery. Chronic fatigue (or recurring shutdown periods, as I call them), frequent urination, and incontinence all started to affect my performance at work. The Premarin did little, if anything, to control the flushes and night sweats that prevented me from getting a good night's sleep. As a result, I felt tired and irritable all the time. I noticed that the flushes grew more severe when I was exposed to high stress levels at work or at home. I also suffered from anxiety attacks that rendered me helpless and led to deeper depression. Why was I feeling so awful?

Connecting with a Good Doctor

Finally, in 1995, I started seeing a family physician whose concern for my well-being was, and still is, genuine. Her plan of action was to help me take care of the weight problem, which would, in turn, take care of the depression. It took more than a year before I could be weaned off Prozac and the daily dose of Premarin could be decreased from 3 to 0.3 milligrams.

My doctor and I found that the minimal dose of Premarin did not appear to cause any additional weight gain, provided, of course, that

I never satisfied my hunger. If I followed a careful eating program, I could maintain my weight. In order to lose weight, however, I had to eat a thousand or fewer calories a day. Unfortunately, this level of deprivation only fuelled my depression.

It was obvious that dieting and power walks weren't helping me shed the post-hysterectomy pounds, so I hired a personal trainer to help me lose some weight. I started doing more cardiovascular exercises, jogging like a fool on my treadmill for the better part of a year until my right knee gave out, requiring surgical repair. I was almost relieved to drop out of my exercise program. Pumping iron was turning my fat into undesirable muscle mass in my arms and legs. I felt and looked like a wrestler, and I still wasn't losing weight. In fact, I was gaining! My weight continued to fluctuate between 158 and 169 pounds. When I lost my job in January 1997, following a third knee surgery, I became so depressed that I actually did lose a few pounds. Unfortunately, the lost weight found its way back to my hips and belly once I recovered, a few months later, from the unexpected blow.

I was suffering more and more from generalized fatigue, poor bladder control, and incontinence, and the severe flushing was beginning to take its toll. I was due for a change in lifestyle. I decided to start a small, home-based writing and editing business. Then I would be able to stay at home and flush to my heart's content without embarrassing myself. I could go to the bathroom every fifteen minutes without raising anyone's eyebrows. Best of all, I wouldn't have to pretend to be happy when I was depressed. I could let the dark clouds roll in and do their thing, and then I could resume my work once I felt up to it. It seemed like the ideal solution. Though networking for clients was stressful, I picked up a bit of work here and there and earned a few dollars for my efforts. I also took some courses in medical terminology at a local business college. The weekly exams triggered so much flushing, I didn't think I'd make it through them, but I did.

I decided to stop dieting; it had become pointless and depressing. Instead, I chose to eat sensibly. There would be no more going to bed hungry and waking up starving. Pushing myself to the extent of risking a fourth knee surgery would no longer be a part of my routine. I began walking for an hour or more every day, and continue to do so. Because I was working from my home office and saw very few people, I no longer had to explain to co-workers why I had changed so much. I found comfort in that.

The transition from a full-time job (and a regular paycheque) to self-employment has been difficult, but I have learned to accept that I am no longer capable of working a nine-to-five day without aggravating my symptoms. I create my own work at home, where the air is cool all year round.

The Turning Point

On January 15, 1998, I was watching *The Oprah Winfrey Show*. The subject that day was sexual desire. When I heard one guest, a hysterectomized woman, talk about her permanent loss of desire, I was shocked. I had taped the show, so I watched it a second time. Then I started pacing, going outdoors into the sub-zero weather to cool down, and then back indoors to pace some more. I watched the tape a third time with my husband when he came home from work that evening. We didn't talk much during dinner, but the program opened the door for future discussions about my lack of sexual desire, a subject we had been ignoring for a long time.

In the months that followed, I viewed several other programs and read a great many books on hysterectomy and related subjects. The CBC's *Marketplace* aired a segment on the dangers of hysterectomy on January 27, 1998. Some specialists, the program reported, believed that North American doctors perform too many unnecessary hysterectomies. One specialist who was interviewed said that hysterectomy brings with it the danger of depression, early menopause, decreased sex drive, and other psychological problems. Finally, I had proof that my problems weren't all in my head.

Armed with this wealth of information, I decided to call the chief of surgery who had given approval for my hysterectomy. I wanted to ask him why I hadn't been told about the many risk factors involved. He told me, "There is no doubt that hysterectomy and ovary removal means instant castration." And, according to him, nothing much could be done to help me now.

Devastated by his dismissal of my concerns, I decided to file a complaint with the Ontario College of Physicians and Surgeons. The basis of the complaint was lack of informed consent. I hoped to raise awareness of the problems faced by the large numbers of women who undergo hysterectomy. Certainly, the specialists involved in my case had neglected to provide me with all the facts on hysterectomy and ERT.

Getting to the Truth

When the College asked me to sign a release form so they could obtain all my medical files, I inquired about getting copies for myself. I asked Nora Coffey, president of the Hysterectomy Educational Resources and Services (HERS) Foundation,[19] to review my medical files. We concluded that my hysterectomy had indeed been unnecessary. Nora explained that, according to the pathology report, all my reproductive organs had been perfectly normal and healthy.

The surgical report provided even more shocking details: "The top of the vagina on the left side was *accidentally entered* during this procedure. For this reason, the vaginal walls were taken with Kochers [clamps] on the left side, while the Heaney clamp was applied on the right side." (I would later read in a medical textbook that Heaney clamps "should not be used in abdominal hysterectomy" because of their crushing force.[20]) The report didn't indicate the extent to which my vaginal walls

19 The Pennsylvania-based HERS Foundation (www.hersfoundation.com) is the only not-for-profit organization in the world dedicated solely to providing education about hysterectomy. For years, Nora W. Coffey, president of the HERS Foundation, has been committed to helping hysterectomized women cope on many levels. See page 199 for more information on the HERS Foundation.
20 Rock, John A., M.D., and John D. Thompson, M.D., Editors. *Te Linde's Operative Gynecology: Eighth Edition.* (Philadelphia: Lippincott-Raven, 1997), 213, 277.

were clamped back, but from the difficulty and pain I had experienced when my husband and I tried to resume sexual relations after the hysterectomy, the adjustment had to have been significant.

The details of this surgical error took on more importance when I found that my family physician and the chief of surgery had neglected to include this information in the patient files I requested from them. In his response to the College, the gynecologist explained away his surgical error in the dismissive style that had become all too familiar to me:

> I read the operative report dictated by my assistant. There is no indication of any complication. I believe that my assistant's use of the word "accidentally" was unfortunate. In removing the uterus and cervix, the vagina is ALWAYS entered, and the top of the vaginal vault is then sutured shut. . . . I usually prefer to clamp the top of the vaginal vault largely closed, with just a small gap in the middle. I feel that this is more elegant, and reduces the risk of infection and bleeding. In some cases, because of scarring from previous Caesarean sections or simply because the cervix is very wide, it is difficult to "feel" exactly where the cervix meets the vagina, and one enters the vagina "accidentally," one bite sooner than expected. This is NOT a complication, and does not cause any problems that would affect a patient's sexual response.

I wanted to tell him that it *does* matter if one enters the vagina one "bite" too soon. I wondered what one or two "accidental bites" represented in inches. In my case, it was enough to seriously hinder my ability to have a healthy and complete sex life. I would have much preferred a less "elegant" procedure that left my vagina intact.

In January 2000, I saw another surgeon for vaginal reconstruction surgery. After conducting an internal examination, he told me that a clump of tissue remained stitched to the top left side of my vagina, at the exact location of the accidental perforation during my hysterectomy. He also noted a lot of scarring along the left side of the vaginal canal. According to this doctor, vaginal reconstruction would be a "tricky" operation, and he could not guarantee that it would correct my sexual dysfunction.

In their reports to the College, my family physician and the chief of surgery were just as dismissive as the gynecologist in their views that there are no side effects to hysterectomy and ERT. The submission prepared by the gynecologist was by far the most arrogant:

In my experience, mastalgia associated with ERT is rare except in older women who have been estrogen-deficient for many years. There is no evidence that ERT increases the risk of breast cancer any more than the estrogen normally produced by the ovaries prior to menopause. [Author's note: The warning labels on any form of estrogen clearly indicate the risk of breast swelling and tenderness, and the risk of breast cancer.]

In my experience, a large majority of women undergoing hysterectomy and oophorectomy report no significant decrease in libido. Many notice improved libido because they no longer have to worry about unplanned bleeding, PMS, pregnancy or pain. A few report a dramatic loss of libido shortly after removal of the ovaries. Most of these respond promptly to testosterone supplementation. Human libido is a complex subject, but I think it is fair to say that the brain plays a major role in human sexual function.

It is hard to believe that a gynecologist with more than twenty years' experience could have so little knowledge about the side effects of estrogen, a drug he prescribed regularly, if not daily, given his medical specialty. However, I found his final remark on human sexual function even more insulting. Telling a patient that her sexual dysfunction is all in her head is not an acceptable diagnosis. I have come across many studies on sexual dysfunction following hysterectomy. One of these, the Wulf H. Utian *Study on the Effect of Hysterectomy, Oophorectomy and Estrogen Therapy on Libido*, for instance, dates back to 1975. Sexual dysfunction in hysterectomized women is not a new phenomenon.

Most surprising was that all three of the doctors stated in response to my complaint that the reason for my hysterectomy was PMS, not endometriosis, as my GP had originally diagnosed and for which my gynecologist had prescribed Zoladex. I know now that the reason for this claim is that the pathology report revealed my reproductive organs to be normal and healthy, and that I didn't have endometriosis. They had to agree on another indication for my surgery.

Our medical system is seriously flawed if doctors believe that castration is an acceptable treatment for mood swings. Even medical textbooks concur. In *Te Linde's Operative Gynecology*, PMS appears under the heading "Inappropriate Indications for Hysterectomy":

> Patients may be extremely uncomfortable with premenstrual syndrome (PMS) symptoms. However, most of these symptoms are related to the ovarian cycle and cannot be relieved by hysterectomy. [Researchers] found only a small improvement in symptoms of PMS in most women following hysterectomy and concluded that neither the presence of the uterus nor the occurrence of menstruation are necessary for the manifestation of the premenstrual tension syndrome and support the view that it has a hormonal basis.[21]

My complaint was dismissed by the College. I appealed. In August 2000, Paul and I appeared before the Health Professions Appeal and Review Board in Toronto. This time, my gynecologist's lawyer presented another theory to explain the accidental perforation of my vagina. According to him, there was no error; the resident who dictated the surgical report was a Francophone doctor who apparently had great difficulty with the English language, and had not meant to dictate "accidental." I pointed out that the French word for "accidental" is *accidentel*, and that there were no other significant grammatical or spelling errors in this very technical report. The Board, however,

---

21 Rock, John A., M.D., and John D. Thompson, M.D., Editors. *Te Linde's Operative Gynecology: Eighth Edition*. (Philadelphia: Lippincott-Raven, 1997), 783–84.

accepted the gynecologist's new explanation and dismissed my appeal. Up to this point, the resident who witnessed and wrote about the surgical error that caused my sexual dysfunction was not questioned.

A recent annual report of the Ontario College of Physicians and Surgeons shows that of the 4,523 complaint investigations handled in 1997, 19 were forwarded to the College's discipline committee and the licenses of only 2 doctors were revoked between 1996 and 1997. Although we have yet to see major changes in policy for this self-regulating body, the provincial Ministry of Health finally did hire a consulting firm to tackle the controversial subject of how well the College handles complaints from patients and disciplines its own members. When this report was released in the spring of 2001, the headline in the paper read "Doctors' Regulatory Body out of Touch."

The Ongoing Search for Better Alternatives

I am still experimenting with HRT in order to find a combination that works for me. I have searched extensively to find an endocrinologist willing to monitor my progress on natural compounded hormones. I tried Prometrium, a natural micronized therapy that mimics the progesterone my body used to produce on its own, but it caused shooting pains in my head, neck, and shoulders. My breasts became very hard and sensitive to touch, and I had migraines so intense that it hurt to run my fingers through my hair. The EstraDerm patch produced many of the same results. Since then I have experimented, with the support of my family physician, with different doses and types of patches. I am grateful that she has not yet given up on me.

In my search for an endocrinologist, I connected with an internal medicine specialist with a background in pharmacology and hypnotherapy. Though I was able to see this fine doctor on only four occasions before he retired, I did learn enough about using self-hypnosis to help myself during anxiety-provoking situations. Finding my inner centre is helpful in regaining control after a flushing episode. It's also a great technique to use when I go to the dentist!

June 1999 was the first time I saw Dr. Alvin Pettle, a Toronto obstetrician and gynecologist and medical director of the Ruth Pettle Wellness Centre. He is one of the very few doctors in Canada to prescribe natural compounded hormones, an alternative to the hormones usually prescribed. Hysterectomized women from across the country come to see him. Toronto is a five-hour drive from my home, but the journey was well worth it. Dr. Pettle diagnosed my shortened vagina and attributed my pain with intercourse to the extra scarring at the top of it, where the cervix used to be. He told Paul and me that nothing much could be done. It wasn't the news I was hoping for, but it did feel good, in a strange way, to get confirmation of what I had suspected all along.

I came home with a supply of the natural compounded hormones I had been reading about and wanting to try for a long time. Three adjustments were made to my daily dose before the intensity and frequency of the flushing and night sweats diminished. I am now more comfortable, though not yet flush-free, and my breast pain has subsided considerably.

I also tried a natural testosterone supplement, a cream applied to the insides of my thighs. It did trigger a spark of sexual desire in me. But, it also caused hair growth on my inner thighs and on my face. One thing I've learned about hormonal therapy is that there is always a trade-off. Before the dark growth on my face could turn into sideburns, I decided to stop applying the cream.

A wonderful American specialist in reproductive medicine further validated my hysterectomy complaints in August 2001. He treated Paul and me with the utmost of professionalism and respect, and there were no deviations in his written report from what he discussed with us following his examination. He confirmed Dr. Pettle's diagnosis, adding that, in his opinion, a vagina like mine, with thickening and scarring at the vault, would have limited function. My surgeon should have used a better technique to preserve the length of the vaginal canal, he said. He told us that there is no remedy for this anatomical defect, and that further surgery would only result in further scarring.

At that point I ended my search for a surgeon who could make me fully sexually functional again. I was sad, but I had a feeling of closure. Maybe it was finally time to move on, and to begin experimenting with intimacy on a whole new level.

One Day at a Time

I am now committed to finding my way back to better health. I try to focus on the good things in my life. About three years ago I started writing a gratitude journal. When I read past entries, I am always surprised at what simple things bring me pleasure and peace.

I continue to be grateful for the loving man in my life. He stands by me, and he can always see the good in me. We share an intimate relationship, one that can withstand change, difficulty, and sorrow.

My boys grew into men before I had a chance to adjust. Each of them has a sensitive side and an excellent sense of humour. I love what they are doing with their lives. They both take pride in their jobs, and I know that they will do well at anything they set their minds to.

I have become ingenious at finding ways to avoid depressive episodes. For instance, there are very few mirrors in my home. If I do walk in front of my bedroom mirror, I do it quickly, and think a positive thought. When I take my bath in the evening (in lukewarm or cold water, of course), I do it by candlelight. It has now become a good way to end the day, rather than a source of further aggravation.

I must admit that I still feel alone at times, and I work hard at trying to forget there was a time when I was a more productive and energetic woman. Looking back makes me sad, because I know that if I had taken time to do the research before I agreed to a hysterectomy, my life would be very different. There is no doubt that my hysterectomy has seriously damaged the quality of my life, and many have noticed the change in me. The surgery transformed me into someone other than the vibrant, gregarious, and productive woman I used to be.

Just before my forty-ninth birthday, I came across a quote on voluntary simplicity:

Voluntary simplicity involves simplifying one's life by choice rather than out of need. It means you put a ceiling on your desires, not necessarily because you have to, but because you want to — you see the wisdom and potential for peace in placing a ceiling on what you want so that you can enjoy what you already have.[22]

It occurred to me that since I have uncovered the truth about my hysterectomy, this is exactly what I have been trying to do with my life. Of course, my surgery is what led me to voluntary simplicity, but lately I have come to realize that what I have is good, despite the menopausal symptoms and the changes in my body, career, and social life. It is this simplicity that keeps my inner spirit alive and well.

---

22 Carlson, Richard, Ph.D. *Don't Sweat the Small Stuff — and It's All Small Stuff*. (New York: Hyperion, 1997).

Beth

❧

I am honoured to include the following story from a woman to whom hundreds have turned for help. In several of the other stories you will notice references to the online forum Sans Uteri. Sans Uteri is Beth Tiner's brainchild.

The first time I saw Beth was in July 1998, when she appeared as a guest on The Oprah Winfrey Show. *The topic that day was "What Women Are Saying About Hysterectomy." After watching, I knew that sooner or later Beth Tiner and I would be talking to each other. Weeks later, we spoke on the telephone, and soon became friends.*

I was moved by the poem she read on the show about the loss she has felt since the surgical removal of her reproductive organs. She was expressing my own grief. I was even more impressed by the organization she founded to provide social support for hysterectomized women and their partners. Without Sans Uteri, many women would not be able to voice the effects that hysterectomy has had on their lives. With Sans Uteri, Beth, and her spouse, Jennifer Russell, we have that voice, and we have each other. (For more

*information about Sans Uteri, Beth's daily structured forum where
people can discuss hysterectomy, refer to the Internet Resources section in Part III.)*

*U*nlike many of the women I speak with, I did not have an unexpected hysterectomy. I consented to the procedure. My doctor
didn't push hysterectomy, nor did he try to sell me on the operation; he
did not "guilt" or frighten me into surgery. I asked him to perform my
hysterectomy after seven years of mind-blowing pain from endometriosis.
At that point I had tried every other option I knew of in an attempt to
stop the pain. Hysterectomy was my final resort.

In February 1987, after seven years of pain-free, healthy menses (I
occasionally took an Aspirin for light cramps), I started experiencing
gut-wrenching pain at the start of each period. I was studying at the
time, and when I returned home from school for Easter break, I saw an
obstetrician/gynecologist who thought that my symptoms sounded like
endometriosis, which my mother had. Even outside the uterus, implants
of endometrial tissue continued to bleed each month. This disease, he
suggested, was probably the source of my pain. That day I started on
the first of many different types of birth control pills, which were supposed to help regulate my cycle and give me some relief.

Unfortunately, the four or five different types of birth control pills
I took gave me no relief whatsoever. Exercise, diet change, pain medication, homeopathy, and herbal remedies didn't help either. For forty-eight
hours a month, I simply gutted it out, taking as much of the painkiller
Darvocet as I could, holding a heating pad to my belly until I burned,
clutching ice until I froze, sitting on the toilet because I could not hold
in urine or stool, vomiting in the sink or shower, clawing at my face
because I felt like I had bugs crawling on me, gasping for air because the
pain radiated down into my thighs and up into my ribs, and begging my
spouse for a knife to kill myself. I felt humiliated because I was missing
work. I knew that "all women have menstrual cramps." Why couldn't
I handle mine?

In May of 1993, I developed shingles. In June, the endometriosis pain, which by now was starting during ovulation, did not stop when my menses ended. One night I called my mom at four in the morning, telling her I couldn't breathe, and that I thought I should kill myself because I just couldn't stand the pain a minute longer. After that, I finally went to my general practitioner, who sent me to an obstetrician/gynecologist, who ordered an ultrasound.

The ultrasound revealed the probable source of my pain: endometrial tissue had grown in my left ovary, creating a benign tumour that was fifteen centimetres wide at its widest point. I was surprised that my left ovary was affected, because the worst of the pain had always been on my right side. At the same time, I was relieved to know that my doctor didn't think my pain was imaginary. Later that month, I had a partial oophorectomy to remove the tumour, leaving me with one intact ovary and one ovarian "stump."

I could have opted for a total abdominal hysterectomy and bilateral salpingo-oopherectomy — in other words, removal of not only the distended ovary but also my uterus, Fallopian tubes, and remaining ovary. But I wanted to put off this radical step for as long as possible, even avoid it altogether if I could. That was part of the reason I just toughed it out each month. I had been learning about endometriosis through the Endometriosis Association since 1987. I knew that many women chose hysterectomy, and that many doctors recommended it as one method of treatment for the condition. I also knew some women were very happy with their hysterectomies. However, through the Hysterectomy Educational Resources and Services (HERS) Foundation, I discovered how much could go wrong, and how much was unknown about the long-term effects of the operation.

So concerned was I about the potential risks and side effects of hysterectomy that I agreed to six months of Lupron injections immediately after my oophorectomy. Lupron is a drug that, simply put, induces temporary menopause by blocking estrogen production. Since menopause puts an end to endometriosis, Lupron can cause the endometrial tissue inside and outside the uterus to atrophy. Unfortunately, it can have a number of unpleasant side effects, and the endometriosis can come back immediately after you stop taking the drug. Still, I hoped that Lupron would give me some relief from the endometriosis, even if only temporarily. I also agreed to try it because I wanted to be able to look back and say, "I did everything I could at the time to stave off hysterectomy with all the knowledge and the strength I had."

My doctor thought a week or two would pass before I began to feel any side effects from Lupron, but I had my first hot flash (the first of many that would last more than twenty minutes) within twenty-four hours of my first injection. Still healing from my abdominal surgery, I began experiencing extreme hot flashes all day and night sweats all night, which meant that I got no sleep. My Lupron experience also included severe joint and bone pain, terrible forgetfulness, and a cold that turned into pneumonia two days after I first noticed a sore throat. I felt so bad during those six months that only once was I able to work a full two-week pay period. I missed work constantly, and I was quickly running out of money. I decided that enough was enough, and stopped taking the drug.

Within two months of my last Lupron injection, my pelvic pain returned. It was as bad as ever, and I spent the final two weeks of February 1994 doing what I had done so many times before — clawing at myself, dripping urine and stool, gasping, vomiting, and taking ever-increasing doses of pain medication.

Going Ahead with Surgery

I asked my doctor to perform a hysterectomy, and he agreed that we had reached that point. On March 4, 1994, not long after my twenty-fifth birthday, I had a total abdominal hysterectomy and bilateral salpingo-oophorectomy. I requested the surgical removal of my uterus, both Fallopian tubes, the top half of my cervix, my right ovary, and my left ovarian "stump."

I do not remember my doctor providing me with much advice as to how I should prepare for the surgery. He knew that I had been reading about it for years, and I was in such pain that our only focus was on getting me through the next week, until I could be wheeled into the operating room.

I knew that microscopic bits of endometriosis could be missed during surgery. I knew that I might need blood during the operation, and made two advance donations. I knew that damage to my other organs could occur, and I had a durable power of attorney form completed so that my spouse, Jennifer Russell, could make decisions for me if I was unable to. I also knew that I might die, and I made a list of what I wanted done with my body and my belongings — just in case.

I was extremely nervous before going to the hospital. The day of the surgery, to help keep my mind occupied, Jennifer and I met my mom and a few friends for a very early breakfast at a local deli. Jen and I watched videos the rest of the morning. I gave myself Fleet enemas, and shaved half of my pubic hair before we left. There was no point, I figured, in paying ten dollars for a disposable razor at the hospital and having my entire pubic mound shaved!

I arrived at the hospital with Jen, my mom, and a friend, at two o'clock in the afternoon. My surgery was scheduled for four o'clock, but it didn't get started until seven o'clock that evening. I spent the hour before surgery alone on a gurney in the hallway outside the operating room. I just lay there and cried quietly.

The surgery lasted an hour and a half. There were no complications. I didn't need the blood I had donated, and the doctor felt sure he had removed all the endometriosis.

The best advice about surgery that I received was from a friend who had had many abdominal procedures. A few days before my partial oophorectomy, she told me to get out of bed and walk, and keep walking as much as I comfortably could, as soon as possible after surgery. She explained that post-operative gas pain can be fierce, and that walking would help ease the gas. After my oophorectomy, I shuffled to the bathroom about ten hours after getting back from the recovery room. With my hysterectomy, I got up about six hours after recovery. (In 1999, I had an emergency appendectomy and removal of hysterectomy adhesions; I was on my feet three hours after surgery.)

Hormone Maze

Although I had done lots of research on hysterectomy and endometriosis before my surgery, I did not have a good understanding of hormone replacement therapy (HRT). My doctor had told me that I would need to take just one pill a day — Premarin — for the rest of my life. If I remember correctly, we did not discuss the pros and cons of HRT. On a scale of one to ten, I had a constant "ten" level of pain, and I don't think my mind could have absorbed any downside to the only option I thought I had left.

I wasn't sure that one pill a day would be the answer to my hormonal needs after surgery; after all, the birth control pills I took for years hadn't worked as advertised. Neither had Lupron, which affected me adversely from the start and apparently did not halt or reverse the endometriosis as it was supposed to do. According to the pathology report from my hysterectomy, I had multiple "chocolate" cysts (filled with dark old blood) and endometriosis "powder burn" lesions throughout my pelvic cavity, even though my last Lupron injection, only ninety days before my surgery, should have kept those symptoms in check.

When I discovered that the Premarin vegetarian me was swallowing every morning came from horse urine, I was distressed, to put it mildly. I didn't know, however, that I had other options. I found out a few months after my hysterectomy that my mom, who was in natural menopause, was rubbing a plant-based estrogen cream into her skin each day, and I quickly made the switch. It would be some time before I learned about natural progesterone cream and oil, products that I have been using successfully since the spring of 1998.

The Trade-off

During the first two years after my hysterectomy, I hurt. I was exhausted, discouraged, depressed, and even suicidal at times. I was never surprised, however, that my hysterectomy didn't make me feel wonderful.

My endometrial pain was finally gone, and I was grateful. But other symptoms surfaced. Six months after my hysterectomy and castration, I realized I was no longer able to completely empty my bladder, that touching my clitoris felt the same as touching the tip of my nose, and that I had such terrible vaginal dryness it hurt to walk. I wasn't sleeping through the night and my energy level wasn't coming back. At times my elbows, forearms, wrists, hands, and hips ached deeply. My skin and hair were dry, and I began to lose my temper easily.

I also began to suffer from vertigo. Sometimes, I'll experience a day of dizziness. Other times, such as after flying, the dizziness has lasted up to two weeks, to the point where I can't walk down a hallway without holding on to the wall. Fortunately, I haven't had trouble with osteoporosis; my bone density scans have actually improved slightly since my surgery.

My weight had increased steadily during the seven years before my hysterectomy when I suffered from endometriosis. It shot up much further after the surgery. I used to be able to lose weight easily; now dropping the pounds takes three times as much work.

Because of my research, I wasn't surprised when I didn't begin to feel a little better until almost a year had passed. I wasn't surprised that I had to visit a number of doctors in order to find one who didn't raise an eyebrow when I went off Premarin and started trying different plant-based hormone replacement regimes. I wasn't surprised that few people understood the havoc that migraine headaches were wreaking on my life. They started three weeks after my hysterectomy; after three years, they had escalated from one every few months to as many as one a day, for months.

I don't think I made the wrong decision. The horrendous endometriosis pain I had for so many years was gone. I knew it could reappear in my bowels, bladder, or somewhere else in my abdomen, but my quality of life had improved. Finally, I was no longer tethered to the toilet, and my world expanded to other parts of the house. No matter how much my head hurt, how little energy I had, or how long it had been since I had the slightest sexual thought, I knew I had made the best decision I could with the information I had at the time.

I am still struggling to find a balance between how much special care my body needs and how much I can do to earn a living. I have very little extra energy, and find this extremely discouraging at times. If I don't take my medication religiously, I suffer the consequences. I try to drink lots of water, practise *qi gong*, walk, and stay away from migraine and vertigo triggers. I have tried many types of estrogen pills and patches, two testosterone pills, and three antidepressants. Zoloft stopped my migraines, but gave me night terrors and reduced my very low libido to absolutely nothing. Paxil caused night terrors and didn't help my migraines. I am currently taking Elavil, which has reduced my migraines and given me vibrant, but not terrifying dreams. It also decreases my libido. Some people think I have tried too many things in too short a time, but they have not been as sick as I was for twelve years. If something doesn't work, I don't have time to waste. So I continue to search for solutions.

I have spoken to doctors about some of my problems, but the details I give them depend on their responses. I have stopped trying to convince them that my hysterectomy and castration have changed me, although indeed they have. Instead, I read a lot and ask other hysterectomized women what they have learned and done to help themselves.

Sans Uteri: A Safe Place

I have written that very little surprised me after my surgery. As I struggled first with endometriosis, then with oophorectomy, Lupron, and finally hysterectomy and its outcomes, what did surprise me was my inability to find a hysterectomy support group in Los Angeles. I had been helping women find health information for a few years. I *knew* I was looking in the right places, but I wasn't finding anything. I wondered why, when so many women were being hysterectomized, when so many women's lives and the lives of their partners and children were being radically and permanently changed. Why wasn't there a place to sit down and say, "I'm eight years post-hysterectomy; I've tried every medication my doctor has given me; I've tried to 'get over it' as my friends tell me to do; I've been to psychiatrists; and I *still* don't feel like me — the me before surgery!"?

I wondered how it could be that so many smart, hard-working women were being forced to quit jobs that their bodies could no longer keep up with, and yet few, if any, people were discussing the financial impact of hysterectomy not only on families, but on the national and global economies.

I wondered how there could be group meetings, retreats, rallies, and fundraisers for diseases that only a fraction of a percentage of the world's population would ever get, yet nothing seemed to be getting done to help hysterectomized women. I wondered why we only ever heard about positive experiences (aside from those featured in the HERS Foundation newsletter) — the ones that went "My hysterectomy took care of my fibroids, I was back to running two miles a day within a month, I don't need any hormones, and my sex life is better than ever!"

I knew there really were women who felt that good after hysterectomy and who wished they had done it sooner. I also learned — from the HERS Foundation's 1996 conference — that a lot of women feel different after surgery, and many feel markedly worse. Thanks to HERS, I connected with a woman who shared my views on the need to develop a global hysterectomy conversation. I mentioned the idea to my Internet service provider, 2 Cow Herd, and that was the beginning of my Internet mailing list, a forum I named Sans Uteri.

On Sans Uteri, I can be honest about how deeply hysterectomy has affected my life. I can run down my list of aches and pains, and someone will respond, "I too had that, and was helped by —." I can say, "My brain is just not what it used to be; I forget everything," and have someone assure me, "It's called brain fog, Beth. You're in good company."

Interestingly, I have found that, even on Sans Uteri, people aren't quick to talk about how hysterectomy affects our ability to work. It is one thing to say, "I have no libido"; it seems to be quite another to say, "I am thirty years old, college educated, and, many days, getting the house vacuumed is all I can do. Working at a regular job is out of the question."

Grateful for Life's Abundance

I have been very fortunate to share my life with an extremely patient person. Jennifer has been my partner for more than a decade, and my best friend for much longer. She has learned through trial and error to tell me when my thinking is not clear and when I am picking a fight. She makes sure I have taken all my pills, and she works at multiple jobs to support us. She went with me to all but one of my doctor appointments over the years, and slept on the floor next to my bed in the hospital after my hysterectomy, caring for me much better than the nurses did.

She has been patient with my greatly decreased libido, and has looked after our house, our animals, our finances, and my aching head, seldom complaining and with very little outlet for her own feelings. She lives with the daily "hormone hell" that hysterectomy can create, and she often goes to work on little sleep because I have talked her ear off into the wee hours of the morning. She comes home with a smile, even though she has no idea what kind of mood I will greet her with. Without Jen, I know I would not have survived.

One of the most fascinating things about hysterectomy is its invisibility. From the outside, no one can tell that a crucial part of my body is missing. I can move through the world with my privacy intact. As a consequence, however, people see me as whole, and they expect me to act as if I were. Because people can't *see* my many health problems, they don't expect me to have any.

When I try to explain how I feel, my attempts are often met with "Just get over it." I wish I could "just get over it," but there is no way to put my organs back and make them healthy. So far, there is no way to restore the way my mind functioned before hysterectomy. If I could "just get over it," I would — but not for the people who feel uncomfortable about my hysterectomy and castration, and not for the people who would prefer it to remain invisible. I would "just get over it" because I miss the me I used to be.

Angela

❧

Towards the end of 1993, when I was thirty years old, my husband had a vasectomy. At long last I was able to stop taking contraceptive pills, which I had been on since the age of eighteen. My husband and I didn't want children, but we had decided it was time for me to stop taking the pill, because we were worried about the potential risk of long-term side effects.

Unbeknownst to me, going off the pill would be the beginning of my medical problems — problems that changed my life and that continue today. I began to have irregular, heavy periods, accompanied by pelvic pain and painful bowel movements. I became anemic. At first I put it down to having just come off the pill. After all, I had been on it for years without a break. As the year wore on, however, I knew there must be some other explanation.

Throughout 1994, I visited my general practitioner regularly because of my menstrual problems. I also saw many other general practitioners and had numerous blood tests, vaginal examinations, and ultrasounds, but never got a diagnosis — that is, other than pregnancy. One female

GP asked me if I "felt" pregnant. Her question upset me. Had she bothered to read my medical file, she would have known that I had never *been* pregnant and couldn't have known what it "felt" like. A male GP boldly suggested that I must be having an extramarital affair — how else could I have got pregnant after my husband's vasectomy?

Finally, after acne erupted all over my face, neck, and back, and after still more blood tests, I was told that I was probably suffering from "a little bit of polycystic ovary disease." I was put on a three-month waiting list for an exploratory laparoscopy to find the source of my problems.

However, by December 1994 the pelvic pain had become so excruciating, and the blood loss so heavy, that I could no longer cope. I was at my wits' end. Luckily, I saw a new, female GP who took my symptoms more seriously than the previous doctors had. Within a few days I was admitted to hospital for an emergency exploratory laparoscopy. (Later I found out that my mother had been so worried about me that she had phoned my GP, insisting that something be done. Her sister had died at age thirty-eight from ovarian cancer, and she thought I was suffering from the same thing.)

Post-operative Shock

When I awoke from my surgery, I discovered two drains in my abdomen and an IV drip — not what I expected from a simple exploratory laparoscopy. None of the medical staff would tell me what had happened during my surgery. Only when my husband came to visit were we able to pry some information out of one of the nurses. She said that my exploratory laparoscopy had turned into a subtotal hysterectomy and bilateral oophorectomy — the removal of my uterus, Fallopian tubes, and ovaries. Only my cervix was left intact.

Apparently, the surgeon had found "chocolate" ovarian cysts and Stage IV endometriosis, the most severe kind. I had widespread endometrial implants — on my bowel and bladder, my cervix, and all over my pelvis. Most of them could not be removed. As my cervix was completely stuck down by the implants, the surgeon could not remove it safely, so I was given a subtotal hysterectomy.

The extent of the surgery came as a total shock. I had no previous diagnosis of endometriosis; in fact, I had never even heard of the condition. None of my doctors had mentioned the prospect of hysterectomy or oophorectomy at any time beforehand. I had not given informed consent for these surgeries; I think the surgeon simply assumed that, because my husband had had a vasectomy and because I didn't want children anyway, he could remove whatever he cared to from my pelvis! I had no idea of the consequences of having a hysterectomy and bilateral oophorectomy at age thirty-one. As for surgical menopause, what on earth was that?

The Aftermath

My consultant told me not to take estrogen replacement therapy for a year after surgery in order to allow any residual endometriosis to "dry up," or atrophy, completely. I was told that there was only a 5 percent chance of the endometriosis recurring if I followed those instructions.

My year without estrogen was incredibly difficult because of the severity of the symptoms of surgical menopause that I began to experience. The hot flushes, insomnia, fatigue, depression, and other symptoms were horrendous. I was put on antidepressants, beta-blockers, and tranquilizers to help control my depression. My GP and consultant kept telling me not to worry; all my problems would be completely solved when I could start taking estrogen in December 1995.

After the year had passed, I started the estrogen replacement therapy. Not long after, my pelvic pain returned, along with some bleeding. It soon became apparent that the estrogen was causing the endometriosis to grow back. After an ultrasound to ensure that my symptoms didn't indicate cancer, I was prescribed thirty milligrams daily of Provera to suppress the endometriosis. The Provera, however, caused rapid weight gain, so I stopped taking it after five months. Luckily, the bleeding had stopped by then, but I still had the pain, which gradually decreased as the months passed.

My GP could offer nothing other than estrogen to deal with my symptoms. Left to my own devices, I began a quest to find my own cure. Thankfully, I had Internet access, and I found all the information I needed by joining Sans Uteri, Witsendo, and other women's mailing lists about menopause. I tried many alternative treatments, including herbal, soy, and homeopathic remedies and acupuncture, to name a few, but nothing helped. I felt so desperately alone.

Because hormone replacement therapy didn't seem to be an option for me, I worried about the prospect of osteoporosis, the thinning of bone tissue that can occur when the body doesn't produce or receive estrogen. I had to go to a private hospital and pay for a bone density scan myself. Thank God I did, because it showed that I had osteopenia, or mild osteoporosis. My GP immediately prescribed Didronel PMO to prevent any further bone loss. He also advised me to go back on HRT, so I tried estrogen again. Within weeks, however, I began to suffer from severe pelvic pain, stomach aches, and nausea. I decided that enough was enough, and stopped taking estrogen altogether.

At that point I managed to persuade my GP to refer me to a hospital where trials of natural progesterone were being carried out. After months of waiting for an appointment, I went to their menopause clinic. Unfortunately, the journey was a waste of time. Claiming that I was too young, they refused to prescribe natural progesterone for me, instead offering me testosterone and estrogen implants. The whole appointment was a disaster — a totally humiliating experience during which the senior consultant spoke to me in a very condescending manner. (I have since discovered that this consultant was convicted in 1997 of serious professional misconduct after removing a woman's ovaries without her consent.)

When Will I Get Better?

As I write this, five years after my surgery, I am no further ahead than I was in December 1994. My surgical menopause symptoms are still with me; they include extremely hot flushes and night sweats, insomnia, depression, and weight gain, among others. Recently, I saw a breast specialist because my right breast has increased in size and is now much larger than the left. I am in physiotherapy for carpal tunnel syndrome and pain and numbness in my right arm, shoulder, and neck, one side of my face, and my head. I continue to be vigilant about osteoporosis and am monitored annually by a rheumatologist, who prescribes Calcichew-D3 Forte tablets (calcium and vitamin D supplements).

Over the past five years, I waited patiently, for months on end, to get appointments with various medical consultants. When their advice and treatment failed me, I tried desperately to help myself, again to no avail. To make things worse, my mother, who was also my best friend, died suddenly from a brain hemorrhage in December 1998, at the age of sixty-one. All I feel now is despair, because the one person I could talk to about my experiences with hysterectomy and its aftermath is gone. I miss her terribly.

I can never forgive the surgeon for performing the surgery without my consent. Every day I wake up and ask myself when this nightmare will end. Will I ever feel well again?

Elizabeth

"*E*lizabeth . . . Elizabeth . . . you have to wake up!"
These faint words seemed to come from far away, through a dense cloud. As I attempted to move, a stabbing pain in my abdomen stopped me short. Bleary-eyed, I tried to focus on the person who was shaking my shoulder and calling my name.

Where was I? Who was talking? Gradually becoming conscious, I realized I was in a hospital room, and a nurse was telling me to swallow the pill she held next to my lips. Still groggy from the anesthetic I had received for my abdominal surgery, I couldn't understand why I needed a pill.

"What's it for?" I asked weakly.

"It's an estrogen pill," she answered. "The doctor removed your ovaries, and left orders to give you estrogen right away, to prevent hot flushes."

Even through my thick fog, her answer baffled me. I was confused. I had signed a release for a hysterectomy, but I understood that the rest of the procedure was supposed to be exploratory only. Why did the doctor take my ovaries? How could they have been causing the pain I had been experiencing? Too weak to do anything else, I swallowed the pill and drifted back under the spell of the anesthetic.

More Than I Wanted

That evening, when the doctor checked on me, I asked him why he had removed my ovaries.

"You not only had varicose veins in your uterus," he replied, "but you also had them wrapped around one ovary. So, since you're over forty and don't need your ovaries anymore, I decided to take them out at the same time, to save you from ovarian cancer."

I was incredulous, and too stunned to respond. *What do you mean I don't need my ovaries,* I thought to myself, *when the estrogen they produce is so critical that you have the nurse rouse me from anesthesia to ensure I don't feel their loss?* But I was too sore, weak, and confused to do more than meekly accept what had been done. After all, how could I challenge a doctor? He must have known what he was doing.

The next day, I discovered stitches in my vaginal opening, and I asked the doctor why they were there. He replied that he had taken advantage of the fact that I was already under anesthesia to cut along the length of my vagina and sew it up to make it tighter. If I had been amazed that my ovaries were gone, this new revelation surprised me even more.

"You never mentioned this before surgery!" I exclaimed.

"It's the normal thing to do," said the doctor. "I just operated on a ninety-year-old woman who had a vaginal prolapse because it was stretched. You wouldn't want that in the future, would you?"

So he had decided to take it upon himself to save me from such an experience. How could he have performed those procedures without my knowledge and consent? Before surgery, we had agreed only upon a hysterectomy. We hadn't even discussed removing my ovaries or "tightening" my vagina. Seeking to understand how these things could have happened, I reflected upon the events that had led up to this operation.

My Life Before Hysterectomy

The cramps I experienced during each period were manageable, but the excruciating pains that came throughout the month doubled me over at times. When the pain came while I was driving, I had to pull over to the side of the road until it passed.

During my period, bath towels were the only things thick enough to absorb my heavy flow. When the excessive bleeding started, my doctor tested my estrogen levels. He informed me that, at the age of forty, I was entering menopause, and offered to give me supplemental estrogen if I wanted it. I agreed to try it, hoping it would be an easy solution to my problems. At the same time, he ordered an ultrasound of my ovaries, the results of which indicated that they were normal.

As the months went by, however, my pain remained just as severe and the bleeding just as heavy. When I saw the doctor again, he told me, "The only answer left is a hysterectomy. Consider it."

It was hard to face the thought of another surgery. I knew from having my gallbladder removed seven years earlier that, no matter what the doctors say, recovery time is difficult. As a single mother trying to raise a seven-year-old daughter, I couldn't afford the time off work or the risk of losing my job. I decided not to have surgery, and my doctor and I continued to work with estrogen therapy in an effort to treat my problems.

After three more years of estrogen, however, I was still bleeding profusely and doubling over in pain. I needed relief, so I made yet another doctor's appointment. The blood work he ordered indicated abnormally low estrogen levels, and he reiterated that I was in early menopause. Again, he said that a hysterectomy would solve my bleeding. As well, it would allow him to explore what was causing my pain.

Before submitting to another surgery, I consulted with a female gynecologist to get a second opinion, as well as any possible alternatives. She concurred with my doctor that a hysterectomy was my only avenue of relief, and emphasized how much better life would be afterwards. Feeling as though I had no other options and nowhere else to turn, I finally consented to the operation.

Accepting the New Me

Now, lying in my hospital bed, in shock as to the extent of the surgery, I knew I had to face the reality that the procedures were irreversible. My only choice was to accept what had been done. After all, my reproductive organs couldn't be put back into my body. I rationalized what had happened by assuming that the doctor's solution must have been the right one, and that it must have been for the best.

On the way home from the hospital, I told myself that all I had to do now was recover, and begin looking forward to a pain-free life, free of the inconvenience of trying to work during my menstrual period.

Over the next few months, however, life was entirely different from the rosy picture I had painted. True, the hysterectomy eliminated the excessive bleeding every month. But other changes surfaced, symptoms my doctors had never discussed with me before the operation. First, my pain was as regular and intense as ever, and I still doubled over at times. For several weeks I passed it off, assuming it was part of the healing process. However, as the months passed, this explanation could no longer justify the recurring, crippling pain. Second, I was becoming increasingly depressed, to an extent unlike anything I had experienced before. Finally, I had lost all interest in sex — it had become a waste of time.

Concerned about these changes, I dragged myself to the doctor's office. "My pain hasn't changed," I told him. "I feel overwhelmed by a growing depression, and sexually, I can't respond at all. I'm making excuses to avoid sex, rather than submitting to something I can no longer feel."

"First of all," he replied, "you can't be in pain — I removed everything. Second, the depression could be the result of difficulty adjusting to the loss of your organs. Maybe you should see a psychiatrist."

He then asked how my sex life had been before the hysterectomy and oophorectomy.

"Fabulous!" I said.

"Why didn't you tell me that before surgery?" he asked.

I was amazed. "I didn't have any reason to discuss it. Why should I have brought up something that was working well?"

His incomprehensible reply was, "I guess I should have asked you about it before we operated."

I was too stunned to speak. Is this how I would be for the rest of my life, I wondered — asexual?

The doctor suggested that in addition to taking estrogen, perhaps I also needed testosterone. The ovaries, he said, made about thirteen different chemicals, including testosterone, which accounted for males' stronger sex drive. He gave me a testosterone shot before I left his office.

Back to the Books

In an attempt to understand what was happening to me, I pulled out my college textbooks to read about testosterone. Since ovaries are the counterparts to men's testicles, they do produce small amounts of testosterone. The books confirmed that testosterone is responsible for everyone's sexual drive, male or female. By now, my lack of sexual response was so pronounced that I realized, even though women produce smaller amounts of testosterone than men, what they do produce is essential.

A few days after the testosterone shot I developed a rash all over my body. When I reported this to the doctor, his only answer was, "It's obvious you can't take testosterone. I have no other options available to you."

With my new understanding of the important role that testosterone plays in our bodies, I became discouraged. I would never be able to artificially replace this critical hormone — and I would never recover my libido.

"Standard Medical Practice"

As the weeks dragged on, my depression grew deeper by the day. I became lethargic; I didn't want to leave the house. I even contemplated suicide. Terrified by these thoughts, I called my doctor, begging for help. Maybe what I really needed, he reiterated, was to see a psychiatrist.

"No," I insisted, "it's not in my head. I'm feeling an imbalance in my body; an imbalance over which I have no control."

He had no answer for me. His removal of my ovaries, he said in his defence, was "standard procedure" for all women over forty. As a last resort, he said, he would contact the experts at the local university medical centre about his decision to take my ovaries, and obtain information about any possible help for me. We set up an appointment to discuss his findings.

At that appointment, he reported, "The experts substantiated what I learned in medical school. They concurred that if you open up a woman over forty, it's best to take her ovaries for her own safety, to ensure that she won't develop ovarian cancer in the future." What he had done, he reiterated, was *standard medical practice.* "Would you want to risk developing ovarian cancer in the future?" Amplifying the threat, he added, "By the time women are diagnosed with ovarian cancer, it's usually too late."

As I left his office, I pondered the definition of standard medical practice. In this case, it meant removing perfectly healthy, normal organs out of a misplaced fear that they might become diseased in the future, thereby risking the patient's present quality of life. It didn't make sense. I wished I could go back in time and undo the surgery.

Putting My Professional Training to Work

I was more confused than ever. It became obvious to me that I needed to know more about hysterectomies and oophorectomies and their effects on the body. I went to the university medical centre library, and started reading all that I could about these surgeries and about ovarian cancer.

As I read the technical and medical journals, I was grateful for my education as a clinical laboratory scientist and for my professional training in medical research.

Everything I read confirmed my own experiences. I found studies that proved that approximately 30 percent of women develop depression following hysterectomy. Articles published well before my surgery warned about loss of sexual response following hysterectomies. Again I asked myself why my doctor hadn't discussed these potential outcomes with me. Obviously he had known about the possible loss of sex drive, or he wouldn't have said that he should have asked about my sex life before the operation.

I made another appointment with the doctor to discuss my findings. After reviewing the material, he agreed with their conclusions, but confessed that he didn't know how to help me. Since he had limited formal training in the complex interrelationships of hormones in the body, his only recourse was to refer me to an endocrinologist, or hormone specialist.

With renewed hope, I met with the endocrinologist. We discussed my depression and loss of sexual response. His solution to the depression was to prescribe a different brand of estrogen, combined with progesterone and thyroid hormones. In answer to my lack of sexual response, this new specialist's blithe recommendation was, "All you need is a new man in your life."

I left his office, incredulous. How could he say such a thing? My sex life before the hysterectomy had been fine. I didn't need a new man in my life. *I* had changed; I knew the problem was within me.

By this point, I had made yet another disturbing discovery about my body. One whole side of my vagina was numb, a result of the cutting and sewing that the surgeon had performed without my prior consent. As well, I had no control over the pelvic muscles on the same side. I knew that these symptoms would hinder my sex life even if my libido did return.

As more months passed, it became obvious that the endocrinologist's new hormone therapy was not lifting my depression. I found it increasingly difficult to go to work. My daily routine consisted of forcing myself out of bed, moving to the couch, and lying there all day, watching television. Even reading, one of my passions, no longer interested me.

I wanted only to hibernate, and began refusing all invitations to socialize. My lifelong friends, whom I loved dearly, just irritated me. The depression felt like a chemical change over which I had no control, and nothing I did made any difference. I felt caught in a downward spiral, falling deeper and deeper into a black hole, with no ability to climb out.

After a year and a half, the doctors gave up on me. Repeatedly their only answer was, "It must be all in your head. You really need to see a psychiatrist."

Hope

Lying on the couch on yet another of my lethargic days, clicking the television remote control, I happened upon *The Phil Donahue Show*. His featured guest was a female gynecologist who described the symptoms of hormone loss that can result from hysterectomies and oophorectomies. As the list of symptoms scrolled down the screen, I realized that almost every one matched those I had experienced ever since my surgery. I could barely contain my excitement.

At last, here might be someone who understood what I was going through! If other women were also experiencing these symptoms, maybe there was some hope after all. I knew I had to see this doctor, and would have gone anywhere to do so. Fortunately, her office was only an hour's drive from my home.

When I dragged myself in to see her three weeks later, she didn't find my description of life after hysterectomy at all surprising. The amount of testosterone produced by the ovaries differs with every woman, she told me. She guessed that I had been a high testosterone producer, and that I was feeling that loss even more than the estrogen loss. When I told her about my allergic reaction to the testosterone shot, she explained that testosterone must be combined with estrogen to prevent women from reacting. Since my estrogen levels were still well below normal, even with estrogen supplements, she said that I obviously wasn't absorbing the oral estrogen.

Next, she asked if my blood pressure had always been high. I explained that on my first visit to the surgeon after my hysterectomy, I was shocked when he warned me that my blood pressure was "dangerously high." I had never had high blood pressure. It has always been so low that doctors and nurses consistently remarked upon it and said how lucky I was. How could I have suddenly developed high blood pressure? The surgeon's only answer had been, "I don't know why, but from now on, we'll need to monitor you closely."

When I relayed this information to the doctor, her reply sent me reeling. High blood pressure isn't uncommon after a hysterectomy, she told me. The uterus secretes a chemical involved in blood pressure regulation, and its loss was probably responsible for my new high pressure. This answer finally clarified a conundrum that had been mystifying me since my surgery.

The doctor gave me a shot of testosterone combined with estrogen, as well as a shot of vitamin B complex. She also prescribed natural progesterone to be taken ten days a month, and a dietary supplement of amino acids.

Returning to my car, I felt like I was walking on air — at last, a doctor who understood what I was going through! She had treated and helped many women with similar experiences. She said she wouldn't give up until she found the right combination of hormones to alleviate my symptoms. Her answers made logical sense, considering that my body was missing pieces of its complex, interdependent chemical structure. Driving home, even with the discouraging news about my high blood pressure, I felt the first hope I had known since my surgery.

Like a Miracle

Over the next several months, as we attempted to restore me to as close to "normal" as possible, my new doctor tried varying levels of hormones, as well as different methods of delivering them into my body. At first, nothing worked consistently. We ruled out oral estrogen because I wasn't absorbing it. Skin patches didn't work well either. Weekly shots of testosterone and estrogen worked best; they made me feel more energetic and less depressed, and I even had days when I felt like my old self again. However, the shots were logistically impractical because the trips to the doctor's office disrupted the better part of a workday each week.

Three years of living hell had gone by since my surgery. I needed to find a consistent, long-term hormone replacement therapy that would relieve my symptoms and allow me to work full-time. As a last resort, we tried experimental hormone pellet implants. These tiny pellets, impregnated with estrogen or testosterone, are inserted in the fatty tissue of the buttocks or abdomen. Their gradual assimilation makes this form of hormone replacement therapy as much like a woman's natural ovarian function as is artificially possible. As well, the benefits last anywhere from three to six months, eliminating the inconvenience of weekly shots.

After the pellets were implanted, I went home and prayed. My bottom was sore, and I had to be careful about how I sat, but by this time I was willing to try anything. I expected and hoped for the same immediate results I had felt from the shots, but one day went by, then two, without any change. After days three and four, still no change. I was becoming discouraged. So many things, after all, hadn't helped before. It had been hard to believe that such tiny pellets would work. Then, incredibly, on day seven I noticed a difference. On day eight I felt even better, and day nine was better still. I felt lighter, and slightly happier. Could it be? Would I finally be helped? Was it possible to feel like I had before the surgery?

By the end of two weeks, a miracle had occurred. I felt like me, whole again. I was overjoyed. It was so much fun to smile and really mean it.

It was great to be up on solid ground again, instead of at the bottom of a dark pit with sides too steep to climb out.

Sharing My Experience

As I returned to the world of the living, I started talking about what my life had been like for the previous three years. When people heard my story, they told me of other hysterectomized women who were suffering from the same kind of deep, debilitating depression, women who, like me, couldn't make it out of the house. Many people asked me to contact their friends and tell them how proper hormone replacement therapy was helping me.

As I met with these women and listened to their descriptions of post-hysterectomy life, I found that many had symptoms like mine. Several had no relief from acute abdominal pain, and many were frustrated by loss of libido. These women also spoke of symptoms I hadn't experienced: thyroid dysfunction and inability to control their weight. They spoke of additional surgeries to unblock intestinal obstructions created by adhesions from scarring. For some, intercourse had become painful because of anatomical changes created by the surgery. Others had experienced hip damage so severe that the simple act of walking had become excruciating.

Hearing about these new problems inspired me to conduct a broader search on the potential consequences of hysterectomies. I was shocked as I began to discover that all the symptoms that I had experienced or heard of had been appearing in medical journal articles for almost half a century. My horror grew as I found thousands of articles, all verifying what these women were telling me. Hysterectomy and oophorectomy have a huge range of debilitating and often devastating side effects, which are well documented in medical literature. Our symptoms weren't "just in our heads." We didn't need psychiatrists; our doctors recommended them out of frustration because they didn't know what else to do.

Based on my research, I filed a complaint with the California Medical Board. After months of waiting, I received the following brief written response: "After our review of your file, we found that the doctor followed standard medical practice in performing your surgery. There is nothing to investigate. THE CASE IS CLOSED."

How could "standard medical practice" destroy a woman's quality of life for three years? After the horrible grief of the previous three years, I wanted to warn other women, hoping to save them from blindly accepting "standard medical practice." I wanted women who had had hysterectomies and oophorectomies to know that they needed to take extra care of their bodies for the rest of their lives. So I wrote a book about the biochemical changes that hysterectomies create in women's bodies: *Hysterectomy and Ovary Removal: What ALL Women Need to KNOW*. (See Publications of Interest in Part III for further information.)

Women's ovaries, uteruses, and cervixes are *not* useless after the childbearing years. Removing these finely tuned chemical plants that nature has so brilliantly provided can have immediate — and lifelong — devastating consequences. In order to make a truly informed choice, women deserve to be educated about all the repercussions that can arise from hysterectomy.

Phoebe

❧

My hysterectomy story begins in December 1993, when, at the age of thirty-four, I was diagnosed with uterine fibroid tumours during a routine gynecological exam.

I had never heard of fibroids before then. The doctor explained that they are benign tumours that form in the walls of the uterus, and that they are rarely cancerous. When I asked him what the treatment was, he said that fibroids were the leading indication for hysterectomy. Surprised that a benign condition could lead to the surgical removal of my uterus, I took home the pamphlet on uterine fibroids he had given me to read, which was produced by the American College of Obstetricians and Gynecologists.

The ACOG pamphlet recommended hysterectomy for women who had completed their families. Myomectomy (removal of just the fibroid, leaving the uterus intact) was an option only for women who wanted to have children. I was confused by the pamphlet. If a myomectomy was technically possible, why couldn't I have one even if I didn't want more children? Wasn't it discriminatory to deny a woman a technically possible procedure on the basis of age or desire to have children?

Over the next couple of years, I didn't think all that much about my fibroids. Although my periods began to get heavier and slightly more painful, I could live with the discomfort. After all, I needed relief through over-the-counter pain medication only one day a month.

In the meantime, my fibroids continued to grow. At a later appointment, my gynecologist told me that my uterus had reached the size it would be if I were eight weeks pregnant. According to him, however, no treatment was required as long as I felt fine. "We'll keep an eye on things," he said.

My periods started to become more painful in the following years. I had excessive blood flow and found that I needed more pain medication to get through the month. Wary of the idea of hysterectomy, I began to research alternative therapies for fibroid tumours. At the library, I found a book written by an obstetrician/gynecologist that described myomectomy in more detail. It sounded to me like a much better option than hysterectomy. I made an appointment with the book's author, who practised in a neighbouring state.

My impression of this doctor began to sour as my husband and I sat for more than three hours in her waiting room. The myomectomy would be rather expensive, so I told her I would have to think things over. My husband agreed that I should hold off on surgery. After all, my menstrual pain was still manageable.

Seeking a Third (and Fourth, and Fifth . . .) Opinion

I saw another gynecologist — my third — for my next routine pelvic examination. When I told him about my fibroids and the new symptoms I was experiencing with menstruation, he ordered an ultrasound. It revealed four fibroids in my uterus, the largest the size of an egg. My uterus was now the size of a twelve-week pregnancy.

I asked the doctor if he could perform a myomectomy, but he recommended hysterectomy, leaving the ovaries. Myomectomies, he said, were difficult surgical procedures that posed greater risk of bleeding and post-operative infection than hysterectomies. Many of them resulted in hysterectomy anyway. If I kept my uterus, he added, I could develop new fibroid tumours in the future.

As the gynecologist was reluctant to discuss myomectomy further, and as I remained unwilling to consider hysterectomy, he recommended that we try a hormonal approach. He prescribed five milligrams of Provera, to be taken daily for the five days before my period. But in a later appointment, he told me that he and his wife used to organize their lives around her menstrual cycle — until she underwent a hysterectomy for fibroids. That comment was my cue to dump him and seek the opinion of yet another doctor.

In March 1997, I saw a fourth gynecological specialist to inquire about alternative treatments for fibroids. I discussed my symptoms and told him that I was still taking Provera. I felt somewhat intimidated by him, but I assumed he had to be a good doctor, since his office was located at a world-renowned medical institution. After conducting an exam and looking at my ultrasound, he suggested that either I try birth control pills or continue with the Provera for another six months. I had read that different contraceptives could cause enlargement of existing fibroids, so I decided to continue with my Provera therapy, even though I was now experiencing severe pain for one day during my period. What other choice did I have?

In the months that followed, the Provera had little effect on my painful and abundant menses. I started passing blood clots. Out of desperation, I tried calling the doctor who had written the book on myomectomy, only to find that she had lost her medical license and moved to another state.

In December 1997, I saw yet another specialist, who claimed that my uterus had grown to the size of a fourteen-week pregnancy. "You need a hysterectomy," he said.

I left his office at a loss about what to do next. I went back to the library to obtain a list of gynecological specialists in my area, hoping to find one who specialized in myomectomy. I didn't find any, and

I couldn't possibly make an appointment with every doctor listed. I pondered my next move. Why couldn't I find a gynecologist willing to perform a myomectomy instead of a hysterectomy?

Just when I thought I had run out of options, a local news program featured a story on a new treatment for heavy menstrual bleeding. Uterine balloon therapy, a form of endometrial ablation, used heat to remove the endometrium lining the uterus. I called the station and was told to contact the ThermaChoice Company to obtain a list of doctors in my area who performed the procedure. I narrowed down my choices to two female gynecologists who shared a medical office. At last I felt I was on the right track.

A Better Life Through Hysterectomy?

My newfound hope, however, was short-lived. The gynecologist said that uterine balloon therapy wasn't an option for me because my fibroids and uterus had become too large. When I asked her if she could do a myomectomy, she said that, while she had performed this procedure, she wouldn't hesitate to undergo a hysterectomy herself if she were experiencing severe bleeding or pain like mine.

I asked her about the possibility of bladder or bowel prolapse following hysterectomy. She replied that bladders and bowels have their own support systems, and added that a prolapse of these organs would be unlikely. When I told her I was afraid that a hysterectomy would hurt my sex life, she said that none of her patients had any problems with sex after surgery, adding that hysterectomy gave her patients a better life. For the time being, she recommended that I take two hundred milligrams of iron a day, because a hemoglobin test had revealed that I was suffering from anemia, most likely because of my excessive menstrual bleeding.

I was confused. If myomectomy was one of the current procedures available for the treatment of fibroids, why couldn't I find a doctor willing to perform one? All the doctors I had seen so far viewed hysterectomy as my best possible option, saying that their patients felt great afterwards. I started to think that if none of their patients had experienced any aftereffects, as they claimed, then maybe I *would* be better off without my uterus.

Approximately two weeks later, in the middle of the night, I experienced what felt like severe throbbing in my uterus. My period had just ended, but my uterus felt as if it were still full of blood, and about to rupture; I didn't feel well the next day. When the symptoms kept recurring, I called the doctor. After we discussed my situation, she refused to even consider performing a myomectomy, and insisted that I needed a hysterectomy.

I managed to get an appointment with the gynecologist at the renowned medical clinic, whom I had seen the year before. I was hoping he might have heard of a new treatment for fibroids since I had been there. After he examined me, he said that there was a lot of pressure in my vagina. He had a surgeon examine me as well. They both said that the size of my uterus ruled out a myomectomy, and indicated that they could perform a vaginal hysterectomy, including the removal of my cervix. I would keep my ovaries, the doctors said, so my hormone levels and function would not change.

When I asked the gynecologist why I couldn't keep my cervix, he told me that it wouldn't do me any good. According to him, hanging on to my cervix would interfere with the healing process following surgery. If, for some reason or other, I needed to have my cervix removed at a later time, he added, the surgical procedure would be very complicated. Finally, he said, the cervix has very few nerve endings and is of no sexual benefit. When I asked about the risk of a prolapsed bladder or bowel, he told me that I wouldn't experience any such problems. (Ten months after the hysterectomy, I developed first-degree bladder prolapse.)

By that time, I was in constant pain. While still terribly reluctant, I consented to surgery. The doctors assured me that I was making the best decision for my health and well-being.

Doing the Right Thing

On October 26, 1998, my uterus and cervix were removed through my vagina. I thought I was doing the right thing in ridding myself of my diseased uterus. I believed that my quality of life was about to improve drastically. After all, why would I, a woman in my forties, want to keep my uterus if it was giving me such problems?

I had no idea what to expect from the operation. With just one or two exceptions, the hysterectomized women I had talked with spoke of a positive experience. All my doctors had provided nothing but glowing reports about hysterectomy, so I hoped I would come out of it okay. Unfortunately, things didn't work out as I had hoped.

No one had prepared me for the dramatic changes that hysterectomy can bring. After my surgery, I became a different person. Things just didn't feel right, either emotionally or physically.

Before surgery, I was active in my children's schools, volunteering as president of the PTA, going on field trips, and helping with reading programs, fundraising, and the school yearbook. I was also involved with a youth hockey organization, a figure-skating association, a gymnastics club, and church activities. I loved going to movies and out for dinner with friends. I helped my husband run our family-owned business. Except for the fibroids, I was happy and healthy in every way.

I used to work out for an hour and a half, two or three times weekly, but after surgery I simply couldn't keep up. In fact, I could barely get out of bed in the morning. I had a hard time falling asleep and staying asleep. Taking a shower became a major undertaking.

I rarely cook anymore; it's too much work. Now my family eats take-out food or something straight out of the frozen food section of the grocery store. I am physically unable to clean our house. I used to be able to focus; now my concentration is no longer sharp. I used to be able to handle the everyday stresses of life; now my emotions are fragile.

After eighteen years of marriage, my husband and I were still very much in love and had a great sex life. Now I feel asexual — my vagina feels strange, I have no libido, and there is no sensation in my nipples.

Penetration is uncomfortable, and my orgasms are weaker, no longer earth-shattering, the way they used to be.

I feel like something is missing. I feel an emptiness in my pelvis where my uterus used to be. I can feel the many adjustments made to my anatomy. My bladder and my bowels are different. Although they were not removed, I believe that my ovaries are functioning at a significantly reduced level. I must now face the decision of whether to take supplementary hormone therapy.

Nothing Is Wrong

Since my surgery, I have had countless tests. Nothing is wrong, all the doctors and specialists tell me. Apparently, there is no medical treatment for my symptoms. Since doctors can't find anything wrong, they have assumed that it must all be in my head. I have been referred to a psychologist and have tried seven different types of antidepressants and anxiety medications. None has been particularly effective, and all resulted in unpleasant side effects. No one wants to acknowledge that the problem is not with my brain.

I am forty years old, and I feel like an old woman. I feel cheated.

Dawn

❦

In 1980, at the age of twenty-three, I visited a gynecologist for the first time. I was seeking relief from a troublesome vaginal infection. Although the doctor's haughty demeanour and gruff bedside manner intimidated me, I was confident in his ability. He prescribed an antibiotic for the infection, but it lingered, so I eventually returned to him for further treatment.

A day or two after a Pap smear, the gynecologist called to say he had reason to suspect that my uterus was "pre-cancerous." He insisted that an immediate hysterectomy was imperative, and resisted answering the few questions my husband and I thought to ask. I didn't know much about the role and functions of my reproductive system at the time, so I placed my trust in this white-haired, dignified, and much-respected gynecologist. We fell in with his plan.

Within forty-eight hours, I was wheeled into an operating room. I awoke stripped of my reproductive system. I had undergone what I now know to be a total abdominal hysterectomy and bilateral salpingo-oophorectomy — surgical castration.

My recovery from the actual surgery was relatively fast and painless. Perhaps that can be chalked up to the resilience of youth. Unfortunately, youth was not enough to absorb the subsequent shock to my body.

At twenty-four, I began to experience extreme emotional highs and lows. The problem escalated rapidly, manifesting itself in manic behaviour followed by periods of complete despondency. I became impossible to live with. A past-due bill, a crying child, or a bad-hair day could provoke an emotional, even violent, episode in me. I screamed at my family and threw things. One Sunday morning, while I was getting ready for church, my curling iron refused to heat up properly. I'd applied my makeup, ironed a shirt for my husband, and laid out clothes for our daughter. Everything was fine until I realized that the curling iron was cold. I completely lost control. My fit of shrieking and crying ended only after I had thrown an expensive cut-glass candy dish through a window. This incident, like many others, was followed by a period of depression during which I could barely function.

My emotional extremes continued for several years before my physical symptoms began to outweigh them. By then, however, my marriage had been irreparably harmed.

Debilitating Symptoms

The first physical symptoms to appear were hot flashes. In the middle of a conversation, I would suddenly feel a flush. Slowly, heat would rise from my lower body to my face. I would begin to perspire, first at the small of my back, then in my armpits, and finally on my forehead and upper lip. When I flushed in the presence of a friend or family member, the expression on his or her face told me that the heat I felt inside was evident outside. A glance in the mirror would reveal a sweaty, beet-red face.

Soon my interest in sex waned. I wanted to want it, but my body wouldn't cooperate. I attributed this latest development to relationship problems, never thinking that it might be a physical symptom resulting from my hysterectomy.

I hadn't seen a physician since the surgery, but the hot flashes finally drove me to my family doctor. He prescribed Premarin, which eliminated the hot flashes completely within a few days. I was profoundly grateful. My interest in sex, however, and my body's response to sexual stimuli, continued to diminish.

In my early thirties, my symptoms worsened rapidly. The mood swings continued. My hair became thinner and dryer, forcing me to periodically adjust its style. Sex began to be not just a bit uncomfortable, but truly painful. I no longer had vaginal lubrication, and orgasm became impossible. I began suffering from one or two terrible headaches a month. After several days of intense pain and nausea, I would often wind up in the emergency room. The frequency of the headaches, which were diagnosed as migraines, increased steadily over the next few years.

In 1988, I separated from my husband. I had assumed that my mood swings, declining sexuality, and general malaise were the results of a bad marriage, or vice versa. It was a reasonable assumption, as the gynecologist who performed my hysterectomy nearly a decade earlier had failed to warn me about the potential long-term physical and emotional implications of the procedure. I had no reason to think that the surgery could have caused all those symptoms.

As my thirties drew to a close, I was still battling severe mood swings. Sex had become unendurable, my hair had thinned noticeably, and my skin was very thin and dry. I sought the opinions of dermatologists, internists, and endocrinologists. All had different suggestions: "Try to eat more protein." "Your depression is causing your physical symptoms. You should get counselling." "Take some thyroid." "Use Rogaine to re-grow your hair." "You're not getting enough exercise." "The headaches are causing muscle tension, and that's making your hair fall out."

Finally, I saw another obstetrician-gynecologist, a woman exactly my age, and a former classmate. My hopes soared; surely, help was on the way! She said I had a dry, fragile, prolapsed vagina, the result of long-term estrogen deficiency. To remedy the problem she doubled my daily dose of Premarin from 1.25 to 2.50 milligrams.

I was reluctant to take such a large dose of estrogen at my age, especially when I thought about my mother's struggle with breast cancer and the link between estrogen and that disease. When I explained my reluctance to the doctor, she said that improving my quality of life was more important than the cancer risk.

My problems persisted, despite the higher dose of Premarin. In fact, they became worse. The long, pretty hair that was once my pride and joy was so thin by my fortieth birthday that I had it cut short — a very low point. By then I had reunited with my husband and wanted very much to enjoy a full, active, and intimate relationship. Sex, however, was still too painful to be possible.

I began to have trouble sleeping. I had difficulty concentrating, and my short-term memory began to fail. I'd always been bright, fast, and efficient, yet I began making foolish errors at home and work. Bills were paid twice, or not at all. Once I left my daughter asleep on the pew after a church service — I didn't remember her until I was almost home. I often found myself searching feverishly for something I was holding in my hand. I had been a reader all my life and dearly loved books, reading at least an hour each night before bed. Before my surgery, I considered it a grand pleasure to curl up with a book and read an entire afternoon away. After the operation, my attention span had altered to such an extent that even that modest pleasure was ruined. I would find myself reading the same passage over and over. Unable to concentrate, I'd soon throw the book aside.

I also developed muscle aches and fatigue. But perhaps the most debilitating symptom was the migraine headaches. They had increased from one or two a month to one or two a week. Neither over-the-counter nor prescription medication alleviated the pain. I began to worry about the vast quantities of pain medication I was taking, but the headaches were unbearable and usually lasted several days, leaving me little choice. Not once did a health care professional suggest that Premarin might be the cause.

Delayed Discovery

Physicians dismissed my concerns. They weren't interested in my hair loss, my depression, or the condition of my skin. The doctors I saw wouldn't acknowledge what I considered to be a very peculiar set of symptoms. I felt like a hypochondriac.

My life was a mess, and I knew I was edging towards a precipice. I was so depressed that I could barely function. I had no sex life, but I desperately needed the comfort and reassurance that a loved and trusted partner provides. I began contemplating suicide. Eventually it became my first thought in the morning and my last before going to bed.

Many doctors claimed that depression was my primary problem and that my physical symptoms were secondary. In desperation, I agreed to see a psychiatrist. He at least took my problems seriously, seeming alarmed at my overall condition. Over the course of several months he prescribed a number of different antidepressants, which had no effect at all. Obviously, instead of psychiatric care, I needed help in overcoming my physical problems. Since no doctor seemed prepared to help, I embarked on my own search for relief.

At the public library and on the Internet, I began to research the long-term effects of surgical menopause. I read about the serious implications of the early removal of a woman's reproductive organs, her primary source of so many hormones. At the age of forty-one, I had been deprived of my ovaries for almost two decades. I was experiencing symptoms common to women in their sixties. I learned that, for premenopausal women, hysterectomy is usually a last resort when all other treatment options are exhausted, and that it should be considered only to treat life-threatening conditions.

I became curious about the circumstances surrounding my own hysterectomy, and contacted the obstetrician/gynecologist who had performed the surgery. He had retired and destroyed his patient records, but I was able to obtain the pre-operative, post-operative, and pathology reports from the hospital where I had my operation. My husband and I went together to pick up the reports, and reviewed them while sitting in the car, still in the hospital parking lot. In his pre-operative report, the doctor briefly discussed his plan to perform a hysterectomy, but provided no reasons for his decision. He didn't mention cancer, and his diagnosis was vague. The post-operative report was not only vague, but confusing.

Tension and dread mounted as we opened the envelope containing the pathology report. It revealed that there had been no cancer, only a mild cervical infection and evidence of an ovarian cyst measuring less than half a centimetre. Nothing more. My reproductive organs had been healthy. Like so many other women, I had been hysterectomized unnecessarily.

We were devastated. We read the reports again and again, unable to believe they could be true. Finally, we drove home in silence.

Finding My Own Cure

I gave up on mainstream medicine and began to search for other treatment options. Initially my search was limited to some extent, because of my conservative and rather skeptical views on alternative medicine. In the end, however, my desperation forced me to learn and explore.

I read a magazine article in which a popular middle-aged actress described her menopause experience. Some medical professionals, she wrote, had been unable to respond appropriately to her needs and concerns. After concluding that estrogen alone, unsupported by other essential hormones, wasn't meeting her hormonal needs, she had switched from standard hormone replacement therapy to a more natural approach.

The actress credited a book called *What Your Doctor May Not Tell You About Menopause*, by Dr. John Lee. I bought this book and several others, and read all that I could about natural hormone replacement therapy (NHRT).

In my case, and for most menopausal women, unopposed estrogen (like the Premarin I had been taking for so many years) is the only therapy offered after hysterectomy. From my research, I learned that progesterone and testosterone are just as important. When I connected with other women like me at various Internet sites (in particular, Beth Tiner's Sans Uteri hysterectomy forum), I noted that many had tried NHRT that included these two hormones, with good results. Even women living with surgical menopause reported significant relief from their symptoms.

I read that many companies manufacture natural, plant-based hormones, such as phytoestrogens, wild yam cream, and others, which are available at health food stores. Compounding pharmacies specialize in more potent natural hormone mixtures, compounded into creams and pills. Although the health food store products are available over the counter, a prescription is required for the stronger, compounded extracts.

I continued to speak to dozens of women every week. All of them vowed that these products had relieved their symptoms. Some reported relief from the milder, over-the-counter products, but most preferred the more potent type.

I set out to convince the only doctor in my area who I thought might listen. Armed with information about NHRT, a list of compounding pharmacies, and a recommendation from a compounding pharmacist I had spoken with, I was hoping he would see things my way.

My husband and I were prepared to argue our view, but much to our surprise and delight, the doctor scanned the materials and said, "I think you're on to something here." He explained that, to some extent at least, physicians rely on pharmaceutical companies to keep them informed about the newest and most effective drugs. Natural products, he said, are derived from natural sources, and thus cannot be patented. For that reason, major pharmaceutical companies have little interest in promoting them, regardless of how effective they might be. He explained that Premarin, the most commonly prescribed hormone supplement, is manufactured by a large pharmaceutical company. That company had done such a good job of marketing its product that many doctors rely on it without investigating other, possibly more effective, options for women. "It's all about money," he concluded.

I firmly believe that this attitude needs to change. Doctors need to educate themselves about the full range of treatments available for women, and not to fall into the mindset that one heavily marketed solution will work for everyone. They need to prescribe treatments that serve the best interests of women — not the drug companies.

My doctor prescribed a sublingual (under-the-tongue) tablet that combined estrogen, progesterone, and testosterone. The tablet was compounded to mimic what my forty-two-year-old body would be secreting naturally, had I still possessed healthy ovaries. I was also given a tube of estrogen cream (natural, of course) to combat my vaginal discomfort.

Within a few weeks of starting my new therapy, my migraines ended. I stopped having hot flashes, sex was less painful, and I began to feel better than I had during the twenty long years since my surgery. I felt more in control of my circumstances, and that gave me hope for the future.

Moving On

Now I know that my symptoms were not the signs of hypochondria or poor mental health. They were the completely predictable and well-documented aftereffects of a hysterectomy performed on a premenopausal woman.

I realize that I will never again feel one hundred percent healthy. The cumulative effects of the surgical removal of my ovaries when I was so young will always influence my physical and mental health, my marriage, and my appearance. My level of sexual function is forever impaired, and I will never again enjoy the intense internal orgasms I experienced when my uterus and cervix were intact.

Perhaps my quality of life will improve even more over time. I hope it will. In the meantime, I am at last in control of my own health care, and I take that responsibility very seriously.

Ellen

❧

In 1966, I took a medical terminology course. As the instructor explained the acronym TAHBSO — total abdominal hysterectomy and bilateral salpingo-oophorectomy — I became very upset when she said that no woman undergoes this operation unless she has cancer. My mother had had the operation five years earlier, and no one had told me she had cancer!

When I pulled my mother's medical records, however, I learned that the operation had been performed not to treat cancer, but because of severe hemorrhaging from fibroid tumours. My instructor had been wrong as far as my mother was concerned, but she had correctly detailed the mindset of that time when it came to hysterectomy: doctors removed a woman's reproductive organs only if they were cancerous. I wonder when things changed. Thirty-three years later, with all the medical advances that have taken place, one would think there would be fewer hysterectomies, not more.

At the age of fifty I began to develop some vague but persistent symptoms: my abdomen was distended and I experienced constant pelvic discomfort. Ovulatory pain would occur on one side of my body, followed a week later by a similar pain on the other side. My periods were very regular, but I had heavy menstrual flow. I had worked for an oncologist in the late 1970s, and I knew that one of the early signs of ovarian cancer is a similarly vague symptomatology, so my own symptoms sent up a red flag.

I spoke to some friends who were nurses. They felt I should take the symptoms seriously and be evaluated for ovarian cancer. I did some research on the Internet — which scared the hell out of me — and then forced myself to face my demons and visit my nurse practitioner. I was actually quite relieved when she and a surgeon in her office told me they thought a fibroid was the cause of my problems.

Pelvic and transvaginal ultrasounds confirmed their hunch, revealing two fibroids and an ovarian cyst. One fibroid seemed to be causing no real problems. The other, much larger tumour was the source of my troubles, which included excruciating back pain that I had been attributing to previous spinal surgeries. To deal with the pain, my nurse practitioner suggested a hysterectomy. I asked her which doctor she recommended to do the surgery, and set up an appointment with him for several days later.

My husband and I met with the surgeon for a pre-op consultation. I had had endometriosis thirty years earlier. At that time, using a minimally invasive laparoscope, a surgeon had cauterized the endometrial "plugs" of tissue that had implanted themselves in my pelvic cavity, and they had never returned. Because of this history of endometriosis, the surgeon felt that the abdominal approach, rather than less invasive vaginal or laparoscopic surgery, was the best way to perform my hysterectomy. By opening my abdomen, the surgeon would be able to ensure that no endometrial implants remained. The anesthesia would be an epidural, as he didn't feel that general anesthesia was as safe.

When the surgeon declared that at my age I didn't need ovaries, my earlier fears of cancer resurfaced; I readily agreed to their removal. He told me that I would need estrogen replacement — "no big deal" — and that I would have no more periods. It sounded so simple and easy.

They Didn't Tell Me

Because my husband would be off work during the last two weeks of the year, we focused only on making sure the surgery would be performed then. I spent little time, if any, researching my upcoming hysterectomy. I refused to allow other women to tell me their horror stories. As with childbirth, I reasoned, everyone has a story, and I didn't want to be alarmed by someone else's bad experience. I have researched new cars and vacations more thoroughly than I researched that operation.

I wasn't a novice to surgery. I had been through many procedures, from laminectomies for herniated discs in my back to rhinoplasty to reshape my nose, several surgeries to remove benign tumours and fibrocystic disease from my breasts, and two laparoscopies, the first to diagnose and treat my endometriosis and the second to remove further adhesions. I knew I would have post-operative pain, but rationalized that back surgery was far more debilitating than any abdominal surgery could ever be. What I didn't factor in was that I had never had an organ removed. No amount of rationalization could have prepared me for what that entailed.

Although I was fifty, I was never told that my fibroids would have shrunk on their own over the next few years as I reached natural menopause and stopped producing estrogen. I was not offered the choice of preserving my uterus by having only the fibroids removed through a myomectomy. I was not told about uterine artery embolization (UAE), a non-surgical procedure to block the blood supply to uterine fibroids, and thus destroy them. I was not encouraged to take a wait-and-see attitude and monitor any excessive pain or bleeding during my monthly cycle. I was not told that my vagina would be shortened when the surgeon removed my cervix, and that the intensity of my sexual climaxes would change.

Actually, I wasn't told much of anything that I now know I needed to be told. I was certainly not told that the person I was on December 29, 1998 — the day before my surgery — would be gone forever.

Post-op

Compared to my previous back surgery, my hysterectomy wasn't particularly painful. Post-operative recovery was relatively unremarkable, except that my blood pressure dropped dramatically several hours after surgery — well below what is considered to be shock. It was remedied by a large infusion of saline through my IV. I was on a morphine pump and IVs, and also had a catheter in place. I didn't sleep for more than a few minutes at a time, which surprised me greatly; I remembered being very dopey after most of my previous procedures. Now, however, when I nodded off, I would open my eyes to find that only a minute or two had passed on the clock near my bed.

Less than twenty-four hours after my surgery, I was sitting up in a chair, waiting for the surgeon to discharge me. All I wanted was to go home. When he arrived, the surgeon agreed to my going home that evening as long as I didn't have a fever and I ate something and had a bowel movement. He gave me some Premarin (0.625 milligrams) and a laxative, and left.

By five o'clock, I was begging to be released. I had no fever, but I hadn't eaten, as I was incredibly nauseated. My bowel sounds were good, and I knew that I would go when I had to — someday. I finally convinced the nurse to discharge me, and went home for New Year's Eve. My only instructions were to return to the hospital if I began to run a fever, started to bleed, or did not have a bowel movement.

I survived my post-op period through trial and error. Sleeping positions were comfortable for only a few minutes, but I did finally get some sleep. I even made the bed, did some laundry, and took care of our pets. At my first post-operative visit, to have the staples removed from my incision, I asked the surgeon if he had removed my appendix, which I thought was standard procedure when operating in the abdominal area. He looked horrified. "No," he said. "Why would I remove something that was healthy?" Indeed — he had just removed two healthy ovaries, two healthy Fallopian tubes, and my healthy cervix!

Post-surgery Changes

The six months following my surgery were a nightmare. I tried to replicate chemically what my body had done so effortlessly on its own. I could no longer rely on it to provide the hormones I needed to feel safe and well. That luxury was lost when my reproductive organs were removed. Whatever hormones they produced, and in whatever quantities, they met my needs. I still hope to find my way through this maze of hormonal imbalance.

I missed terribly the woman I used to be. I knew her well — we had fifty years together. But now she was lost to my husband and me. The person who replaced her was much more unpredictable. Stresses in my life that I could once deal with effectively now caused anxiety attacks or almost instantaneous Jekyll-and-Hyde transformations. If my husband said something to me in jest, I would overreact and get angry at him. Vacations, once an enormous source of pleasure, were now highly stressful. I used to love to travel; now I needed to take an Ativan before getting on a plane. I became much more introspective and high-strung. I didn't know how or why I would react to any given situation; I seemed to have no control over my emotions.

Without any change in my diet or exercise, I gained fifteen pounds over the three years following my hysterectomy. My skin became much drier; I looked haggard, older. I had a history of chronic depression and had been taking antidepressants on and off for years. So, after reading that many women become depressed after hysterectomy, I started taking Zoloft, because I was afraid that I would find out I was depressed, and I didn't want that black cloud hanging over my head ever again.

The Premarin caused six weeks of nausea and anxiety attacks. When I told my surgeon about those side effects, he suggested a gastrointestinal work-up and therapy. But when I stopped taking the hormone, the nausea and anxiety disappeared.

I read about loss of libido, and that surgeons often shortened the vaginal canal when they removed the cervix. When I asked my surgeon if he had shortened my vagina, he answered very matter-of-factly that of course he had — how else could he remove my cervix?

I was terrified that sex would never be the same. Three weeks after surgery, my husband and I experimented to see if I could still have a climax. Tearfully, I found out that I could. Three weeks later, we made love for the first time, and I was relieved to find that, although sex was different, it was still good. It would have been great if I were still able to experience uterine contractions and cervical pressure, but it was still more than I had hoped for.

Support and Friendship

Because I had been given no instructions for life after hysterectomy, I searched the Internet for a site that could help me through my recovery. I found Sans Uteri, and it's thanks to the support, caring, and sharing of the wonderful ladies of this forum that I have been able to manage the transition to the extent that I have. Because of them, I am who and where I am right now.

They gave me advice on what I could do and should not do. They educated me about hormone replacement therapy. They verbalized their frustrations with their surgeons, so that when my surgeon brushed my concerns aside, I wasn't surprised or angry. They gave me the guts to stand up to him and say, "No, I will not take Premarin any more." They recommended books that educated me about post-operative recovery, and armed me with the information I would need to maintain my quality of life in the future. Most of all, they showed me that I wasn't alone in my quest to be the person I once was. (For more information on Sans Uteri, see Internet Resources in Part III.)

Awareness Is the Key

Since my operation, my nurse practitioner has agreed to journey with me in learning about hormone replacement therapy. I now use an estrogen patch instead of Premarin. To supplement my hormonal needs, I also use a cream that has progesterone and testosterone compounded into it. While it works, it still needs a great deal of fine-tuning in order to meet my specific needs. I am learning, the hard way, that every day is a new experience.

I am blessed to have the support and love of a wonderful husband who feels as challenged by this quest as I do. I am also blessed by the encouragement and care of wonderful friends. Many of them I have met since my surgery, but I cherish them as greatly as I do my long-time friends, many of whom are, or may someday be, where I am today.

There are lessons to be learned from my story. Women facing hysterectomy and oophorectomy must be better educated about the various surgical and non-surgical options available to them. Surgeons must consider more carefully the effects of their actions on women's current and future health and well-being. The media need to give as much publicity to this devastating operation as they give to issues like male impotence and computer viruses. "Informed consent" must become not just a piece of paper, but a real awareness of what can and will happen to women who have their reproductive organs removed.

Jeannah

❧

My story begins in mid-1996, when I went to the doctor to explore further treatment options for endometriosis. I had already had two laparoscopic surgeries, one for diagnostic purposes and the next to remove endometrial implants throughout my pelvic cavity. I had tried Lupron, which suppresses menstruation, ovulation, and the production of estrogen, which stimulates the growth of endometriosis. I had tried birth control pills, Synarel nasal spray, and all the non-steroidal anti-inflammatory drugs known to man. None of those treatments was able to rid me of endometriosis, which not only deposits endometrial tissue throughout the pelvic cavity, but also often forms internal scar tissue, or adhesions. In many women, including me, these adhesions can cause great pain.

My endometriosis pain started when I was thirteen, and it had always been severe. Birth control pills managed to keep the disease at bay and the pain under control, but unfortunately, as with all the other drug therapies I tried, the pain would come back immediately after I stopped the treatment or very shortly thereafter. My 1995 laparoscopy had revealed extensive endometrial implants and adhesions scattered throughout my abdominal cavity, along with cysts and other lesions caused by the disease. I was afraid that the endometriosis would spread further, to my bowel and bladder, where it can cause serious complications.

My doctor suggested another round of Lupron. I refused, knowing the potential dangers of this menopause-inducing drug, and that it would bring only temporary relief at best. She told me to think about it, and wrote out a prescription for the drug that I had just told her did nothing for my pain. I sighed heavily as I waited for the nurse to get my prescription. On my way out of the doctor's office, I picked up a pamphlet called *A Woman's Guide to Hysterectomy*. I wondered if the removal of my uterus would someday be my final resort.

During the next eleven months, the endometriosis pain grew worse. My quality of life dwindled considerably. I was symptomatic for three weeks of every month. Excruciatingly painful menstrual cramps lasted three or four days, beginning the day before my period. I was constipated and severely bloated. I had backaches, pain with intercourse, and pain with ovulation that lasted anywhere from two days to two weeks. I took 1200 milligrams of Ibuprofen to control the pain (the dose for an average headache is 200 milligrams). I was going through a hundred-tablet bottle of Ibuprofen a month, and I often thought about buying stock in the pharmaceutical company that made it! The medication wasn't very effective, but it took enough of the edge off the pain that I could function.

Endometriosis will usually disappear on its own when a woman reaches menopause and stops producing the estrogen that stimulates it. I didn't want to wait another ten to fifteen years before I reached natural menopause. I was ready for an end to this painful and destructive disease. Hysterectomy seemed like my only option.

Finding the Right Specialist

By May 1997, I had a new job, and with it, better medical insurance coverage. I visited my primary care physician, who agreed that it was time for me to see a specialist about my endometriosis.

A few years earlier, another endometriosis sufferer and I had organized an Endo Support Group in our area. At the meetings I had heard talk about a doctor, in a town about fifty miles away, who was experienced in treating endometriosis. I knew that finding an experienced specialist was an important part of correctly managing this complicated disease.

I couldn't believe my good fortune when this doctor appeared on the list of providers whose services were available through my new insurance company. I was thrilled. I told my primary care doctor that he was the specialist I wanted to see. The referral was made, and an appointment was scheduled for June.

I waited with great anticipation to see this doctor. As the appointment time grew near, I was filled with hope. Finally, with the help of the new specialist, I would have a solution that could put an end to my suffering. While I was curious as to what he would recommend, by then hysterectomy seemed to be the only option left.

I saw Dr. Z on June 11, 1997. He and I discussed my medical history, as well as all the treatments and surgeries I had undergone in hopes of ridding my body of endometriosis. He agreed that I had tried them all. He asked me if I wanted any more children. I was thirty-six, the mother of a fifteen-year-old, and I had had a miscarriage just the year before. I told the doctor that I had come to terms with the fact that my childbearing days were over. I didn't want to go through the pain and heartbreak of another miscarriage.

Talking About Hysterectomy

The doctor recommended a total hysterectomy and bilateral salpingo-oophorectomy and he also recommended removing my cervix. We discussed the pros and cons of leaving my ovaries and cervix. Because of my long and painful history with endometriosis, I didn't want to risk a recurrence of the disease, or to have the remaining organs removed at a later time. We agreed that a total hysterectomy was my best choice.

Before leaving Dr. Z's office that day, I signed the consent forms for an abdominal hysterectomy, exploratory laparotomy, and bilateral salpingo-oophorectomy. The form included the usual information on the risks of surgery, such as complications from bleeding and infection, damage to other organs, and even death. In retrospect, I think that any consent form for hysterectomy and/or oophorectomy should be required to provide warnings about the effects that can arise from the loss of ovarian hormones. Once a woman's ovaries have been surgically removed, doctors tend to group her with women who are going through natural menopause, and they prescribe the same types of hormonal therapies for them. As I would discover, however, there is a huge differ-ence between the slow, gradual, and natural decline of ovarian function and the instant and complete hormonal loss that sometimes comes with hysterectomy, and always with oophorectomy.

Once I had made my decision, I felt a sense of peace. During the month before my surgery, I signed out all the library books I could find on hysterectomy, hormone replacement therapy, and menopause. Our relatively small library didn't have much of a selection. The books I read provided few details on the complications that can arise following the surgical removal of the ovaries. How I wish now that I could have had some warning about what was in store.

H-Day

On July 17, 1997, my mom and I drove to the hospital. I felt ready. However, it wasn't until I began signing the admission paperwork that it really sank in. This was it.

We arrived at the pre-op room at seven o'clock in the morning, but a nurse came in to tell me that the surgery would be delayed until one o'clock that afternoon. I wondered if I should just go home and forget about it — maybe the delay was a sign. But the time passed quickly, and the attendants came to get me at 11:30 a.m. They were ready and I was ready. It was time.

When I awoke from surgery, I was already in my room, and barely coherent. I was in agonizing pain, which lasted through the night, despite the fact that I was hooked up to a morphine pump. My abdomen felt as though it had been ripped apart. I couldn't get comfortable. My mom and my daughter and her boyfriend were there, but I couldn't keep my eyes open or stay awake long enough to talk to them.

Anxious to be in my own bed, I went home the next day. There was some disagreement among the nurses about whether to give me my next dose of pain medication. However, knowing that I had an hour-long trip ahead of me, I insisted on taking the medication before I left. As soon as it was administered, I hobbled out of there.

A Long Recovery

At home, I was couch-bound for two weeks, and most grateful for my daughter's help. Recovering from surgery is different for everyone. Some women are out playing golf in two or three weeks, but not me! I battled with my normally energetic, take-charge self, reminding myself to take things nice and slowly, and avoiding the impulse to jump up and handle everything.

I have since been told by other women that those who go into surgery with a positive attitude experience a quick recovery. I did feel very positive about the operation. I was at peace with my decision, and I had no preconceived notions about potential negative outcomes. I was eager to be rid of the endometriosis, the pain, and the complications that I had lived with for so long. I was anxious to feel normal again. Despite my preparations and positive outlook, my recovery period was long.

After a week, I began going outside for short walks. My dog was only too happy to get out, but I would start feeling weak and light-headed after walking only a short block. I felt guilty about not being able to walk much, but I simply couldn't do more.

For financial reasons, I had to go back to work after four weeks. I started with just four hours a day, and made it back to eight hours the following week. I felt exhausted, and wished I had been able to take a full six weeks off.

About two weeks after surgery, I began to have bladder spasms and pain with urination. I went back to my doctor, who concluded that I had an infection, probably from the catheter in the hospital. He prescribed medication for the spasms and antibiotics for the infection. The condition improved after two weeks, but much to my dismay, I developed urinary incontinence and leakage.

Six weeks after my surgery, I visited the doctor again. He did a tampon test to get to the root of the urinary problem, to see if urine was leaking into my vagina through a tear or rupture. I was relieved when the test revealed no leakage or infection, and the problem resolved itself in approximately two weeks. The doctor couldn't explain its cause. I suspect, however, that it might have resulted from low levels of estrogen. I have since experienced this condition a few more times, especially when switching from one hormone therapy to another.

The HRT Odyssey

Six weeks after my surgery, Dr. Z's partner in practice, who had an office near where I lived, declared that I was healed, back to normal, and ready to resume my life. We discussed hormone replacement therapy. I had read Dr. John Lee's book, *What Your Doctor May Not Tell You About Menopause*, and a few other books on the same subject, and was leaning towards natural hormone replacement therapy. I believed, as I still do, that the synthetic hormones (birth control pills) that I took to control endometriosis over many years had served a purpose, but I also felt that they probably did more harm than good.

Dr. Z's partner suggested that I should start out on Premarin, but

I was firm in my decision to opt for NHRT. He was less than enthusiastic about my plans, stressing the many benefits of Premarin. He would prescribe it for his own mother, he said. But he didn't convince me.

I had my reasons for wanting to stay away from estrogen. A great deal of the material I've read supports the theory that if any endometriosis is left in the pelvic cavity following hysterectomy, it can be kept alive and active by estrogen therapy. This makes perfect sense to me, given that endometriosis is estrogen dependent. I had only an elementary understanding of HRT and NHRT at the time, but I was insistent, and the doctor finally consented to prescribing Ogen, which is made from estrone, a weak form of estrogen. It wasn't a natural hormone replacement, but I didn't know that at the time.

Unfortunately, Ogen made me feel bloated and irritable. I had headaches and began developing cystic acne. My body was obviously trying to tell me something. Back at the library, I went over Dr. Lee's book again, and decided I should try the natural progesterone cream he discusses. I hoped it would take care of the hot flashes and the night sweats that started some two months after my surgery, and that it would buy me some time so I wouldn't have to take estrogen and risk the return of my endometriosis.

I bought the cream at a local health food store, and started using it twice daily. After just three weeks, the flashes and the night sweats disappeared completely. After more than three months on the progesterone cream, I began to feel more energetic. As well, I began to lose weight without trying, and my libido and mood improved significantly. By December 1997, I truly felt like a new woman — healthy for the first time since surgery, and without the debilitating pain of endometriosis.

In January 1998, I was feeling so good that I decided to decrease my daily dose of progesterone in an attempt to cut down on expenses. That was a big mistake! A word to the wise: if it ain't broke, don't fix it! The hot flashes returned within a month. As soon as I felt the first flush, I upped my application to the original dose, but unfortunately, I think it was too late to undo the damage. By lowering my dose of progesterone, I believe I created the wrong environment for my endocrine system.

By April 1998, I had begun to experience a host of problems caused by the severe hormone loss that occurs when a woman's ovaries are removed. Depression had set in by June, and I started taking the antidepressant Paxil. I had no interest in sex and I was incredibly fatigued. I had short-term memory loss and I wasn't able to concentrate at work. By August, these debilitating symptoms had progressed even further.

Pain in my joints caused me great discomfort. Every day I woke up with a different joint pain. It started in one knee, and then it moved on to my elbow, hip, and lower back. Some days, even my finger joints ached. Muscle relaxants and pain relievers had no effect. I had terrible pains in my left foot, so that I hobbled at work. My doctor's only explanation was that I was overweight and needed more exercise. I had been moderately overweight most of my life, however, and had never experienced symptoms like those.

Finally the doctor explained that it was normal for women my age (thirty-six!) to have aches and pains. But I knew that this intense pain wasn't normal. To help myself, I began taking glucosamine sulphate, a natural joint remedy. I also tried acupuncture, but with little success. I didn't go back for further treatments; it was too painful, and I was already hurting enough.

NHRT, the Option for Me

Finally, I decided to pursue natural hormone replacement therapy. I had exchanged stories and compared notes with many women who had had hysterectomies, and I learned that those who felt best were on NHRT.

I discussed my symptoms with a compounding pharmacist, who recommended a starting dose. It took a while to convince my primary care physician that NHRT was the option for me. After reviewing the literature I brought her, she told me that she didn't know much about the treatment, but if it worked for me, it would make a believer out of her.

I started NHRT in October 1998. My joint pain and other body aches began to subside. I was still fatigued, however, and hadn't noticed any improvement in my libido at the three-month mark, which is the recommended time to stay with one dose to determine its effect. The pharmacist recommended that I increase my dose from twice to three times daily. With my doctor's approval, I went ahead with the more frequent dose.

I also started going for a therapeutic massage once a week. After my unsuccessful experience with acupuncture, I wanted to try something to help me relax and feel good and that wouldn't cause me additional pain. Massage turned out to be a very positive treatment option for me, and it is one of the few things I do just for myself. I find that my weekly massages help me to continue on, despite daily pain.

By January 1999, my spells of fatigue had grown more severe, and the joint pain, stiffness, and other aches had returned. I started taking multivitamins, and I bought a better mattress and an exercise bicycle. I also changed my eating habits.

Unfortunately, the pain in my lower back and left hip remained constant, hampering my ability to walk. It was all I could do to make it up the stairs to my apartment after a day's work. Riding my exercise bike was definitely out of the question!

Trial and Error

I researched other methods of NHRT and discussed my findings and recurring symptoms with any doctor or compounding pharmacist who would listen. Finally, something clicked in my head about the product I was taking. I remembered seeing "MTT" on the prescription label, and I wondered if it stood for methyltestosterone, a synthetic form of testosterone. Sure enough, it did. I thought I had been prescribed only completely natural hormones. Somebody, somewhere, had made a mistake.

Through experiments with different forms of hormone replacement therapies, I quickly determined that my body indeed reacted negatively to synthetic forms of these drugs. When I discussed my situation with an experienced compounding pharmacist, he recommended that I stay away from oral micronized NHRT and try instead a combination of estradiol, estriol, progesterone, and testosterone, all in transdermal (cream) form. When I finally latched on to the NHRT that was right for me, my symptoms began to improve immediately.

These days I feel more like the woman I used to be before my hysterectomy, and my family has noticed the change as well. My joint pains and body aches are less severe. However, I still struggle with fatigue, short-term memory loss, and poor concentration. When I encounter any type of stress or emotional upset, my body reacts negatively and most of my symptoms return. I am committed, however, to staying on my current prescription for one full year. I feel strongly that this is the safest route for me.

I pray that my body and its endocrine system will return to normal. I also hope that research will lead to more effective methods of treating endometriosis and other reproductive diseases — methods that do not involve removing a woman's female organs. I now run a Web site (www.hysterectomyawareness.com) dedicated to educating women about hysterectomy from the perspective of those who have been there. I hear every day from women who have (or had) no idea about the potential health consequences of hysterectomy and oophorectomy. Women and physicians need more and better education about these life-changing surgeries.

Amber

❧

"Pelvic inflammatory disease . . . presents an enormous threat to female fertility, and often the internal scarring caused by the infection can lead to chronic pelvic pain. Hysterectomy may be recommended to relieve the pain. With the advanced surgical techniques and antibiotics now available, however, there is seldom any reason to consider hysterectomy as a treatment for PID."

— STANLEY WEST, M.D.,
AUTHOR OF THE HYSTERECTOMY HOAX

I became ill in May 1993. I had been suffering from a yeast infection, a fairly common occurrence, but this time the infection was causing me greater discomfort than any previous one I'd had. Since it was a long weekend, no medical clinic was open. I went to the closest hospital, where I saw the doctor on call.

The doctor ordered a urine test and took several swabs. I was diagnosed with a severe infection and pelvic inflammatory disease (PID).

I had never heard of PID, which, I would later find out, is an infection of the pelvic organs that can lead to infertility from internal scarring if left untreated. To put me at ease, the doctor explained that he was a gynecologist, and that he dealt with situations like mine all the time. He prescribed antibiotics for both my husband and me, to prevent a recurrence of the infection.

A week later, I still wasn't feeling any better, so I went to the same doctor's clinic, where further blood and urine tests were done. He prescribed more antibiotics. During the visit, I mentioned that I had recently had a bladder infection. I asked the doctor what was causing the infections and what I could do to get rid of them. He asked about any other symptoms I had, and I told him about my heavy periods. He suggested healthier eating habits and exercise to strengthen my stomach muscles. When I asked him what else I could do, he asked if I had ever considered having a hysterectomy.

I was only twenty-eight years old. No doctor had ever mentioned hysterectomy to me. But this gynecologist began to insist that removing my uterus would be the best thing I could ever do. He stressed over and over the importance of ridding myself of PID. He asked my husband, who was sitting in the waiting room, to come in to hear how hysterectomy would make a new woman of me. I would have no more periods, no more pain, and no more infections. At last he convinced me that hysterectomy was my only option. The surgery was booked, and I was to have a hysterectomy less than a month later.

I don't know why sirens didn't go off in my head, because my husband and I did have concerns about the operation. Our greatest distress was that we wouldn't be able to have children. We weren't particularly worried about the health risks, however, because the doctor minimized them in his glowing description. We thought highly of the doctor and his advice, and we trusted him completely. And any doubts or fears I had were put to rest once I saw my family physician, who concurred with the gynecologist's recommendation that I undergo the hysterectomy.

On June 26, I went back to the gynecologist's office to complete the forms for my surgery, which was scheduled for the following day. The doctor explained that he wouldn't remove my ovaries unless they were unhealthy or diseased. I told him clearly that I did not want them removed. After all, I thought, I was too young to go through menopause. I didn't know much about PID, but I knew enough about menopause to be sure that I wanted to delay it for as many years as I could.

The next day, just three weeks from the day I first met the gynecologist at the hospital, I had a total abdominal hysterectomy and bilateral salpingo-oophorectomy. I didn't find out about the oophorectomy until two days later.

Feeling the Pain of a Surgical Error

During the three days following surgery, I felt sick. I was pale, I had severe abdominal pain, and I had difficulty voiding urine. Nurses and family members told me that these symptoms were normal following major surgery, and that I would feel better soon. I was in too much pain to find comfort in their words.

I was released from the hospital on the third day, but I was in so much pain that my mother brought me back again that night. I still couldn't void, and it really hurt. After I had waited in agony for several hours, the gynecologist finally arrived. He gave me an injection of Demerol and other medications for the pain, and inserted a catheter. I felt a lot better after that. Finally, I could empty my bladder.

The doctor was reluctant to readmit me to the hospital; he claimed that it would be difficult to find a bed for me. I insisted. I knew my hospitalization was justified, but the nurses treated me very poorly. Some said my problems were all in my head. Others said that if I just sat up and relaxed, I would be able to void. Another told me that most women who undergo hysterectomy get up and walk a lot sooner than I did. I was stunned by their cruelty.

I felt deathly ill for the six days following my hysterectomy. The abdominal pain was unbearable, and I required injections of Carbachol to void, Demerol to control the pain, Gravol to control the nausea, and Valium and Ativan to help me both void and relax. I developed another infection. My catheters had to be constantly removed and reinserted.

My blood count dropped with each passing day, but no one reacted to that until the doctor finally ordered an intravenous pyelography (IVP), an X-ray of the kidneys and ureter. Before the test, I was given a double dose of drugs to help me urinate. They provoked a sensation that I needed to void, but I still couldn't go. My frequent trips to the bathroom seemed to irritate the nurse, who wanted me to lie still for the X-ray. She made me feel that my pain and symptoms were all my fault.

Shortly after the test, and six days after surgery, a doctor came in to see me. He reported that my problem was caused by a blockage of some sort, and that I would be sent to another hospital the next day for a cystoscopy and a cystogram, tests to examine my bladder and urinary tract. I was asked to provide my own transportation for those additional tests, after which I was to return to the hospital.

The next morning, there was a change of plans. The hospital I was being sent to could not perform the required tests, and the doctor made arrangements for me to go to another one — this time, by ambulance. The ambulance drivers had said that they would be back to pick me up in a few hours, but the woman at the admissions desk told me I was being admitted. When I replied that I had been brought in for tests only, she still insisted that I fill out the necessary admission forms.

Apologies

After the cystoscopy, the doctor who performed the test came over to see me. He said that my bladder had been perforated during my hysterectomy, and I would have to undergo emergency surgery to repair it. They wheeled me into the hospital corridor. I began to cry as I sat there alone. Why was this happening to me? My only consolation was that the diagnosis meant my symptoms hadn't been imaginary after all.

I was immediately prepped for surgery. I didn't have time to contact my family, and I was scared. As I was wheeled into the operating room, I grabbed at a nurse, begging her to call my family and let them know I was having another operation.

I must admit that I did feel better after the second surgery. Everyone said I looked a hundred percent healthier. When I finally had a chance to talk to the surgeon who repaired my bladder, he explained what had happened. Because of the perforation in the bladder, urine was leaking into my abdomen and poisoning me. When I asked him how big the hole was, he held together his thumb and forefinger to show me — the tear was as big as a one-dollar coin! Because of the blockage, he had had to cut open my bladder and drain it of several hundred cubic centimetres of urine. At one point during the surgery, he had even thought I might need a blood transfusion.

As I recovered from my emergency surgery at the second hospital, the gynecologist who had performed my hysterectomy came to see me. He apologized for what I had been through, and admitted that it was all his fault. Nothing like that had ever happened to him, he added, and he could not understand how my bladder had been perforated to that extent.

He went on to explain that he had used a special clamp with which he had not had much experience, but the representative from the company that made the clamp had been in the operating room to guide him. At that point my husband and I forgave him. Again he apologized profusely, and kept repeating that he felt awful. It was hard for me to respond. Finally, the gynecologist said that he wouldn't use the new clamp any more. (Much later, I would find out that he had lied. He didn't use the clamp, and no one from the company had been with him.)

As for removing my ovaries, the gynecologist said he had no choice in the matter. One of my ovaries was apparently attached to my side, while a cord had somehow wrapped itself around the other. I felt numb as I watched him leave the room.

Going Home

I stayed in the second hospital for six days. On the morning of the day I was to be released, the surgeon removed the catheter inserted just above my pubic hairline. All I needed to do was void once, he said, and I could go home. That sounded simple enough. A few hours later, however, urine came pouring out of me like water from a tap!

I told the nurses that couldn't be normal, but they insisted it was. They took turns bringing in bags of sanitary pads and gauze. Some of them joked about putting a cork in me to stop the urine coming out. After they had twice replaced the sterile strips on my incision, one nurse said there was no point in applying others, because the urine would only dampen them, too. At one point I asked a nurse to call the surgeon to get his view of this new problem, but she replied that he was already aware of my situation. I was released from hospital with a stack of four sanitary pads bunched between my legs to absorb the unstoppable flow of urine.

When I got home, my husband decided to call the gynecologist who had performed my hysterectomy. The gynecologist agreed that my predicament wasn't normal, and said that he wanted to see me as soon as possible. I couldn't believe what I was hearing! The doctor who had ruptured my bladder was the last person I wanted to see, but my husband insisted.

My mother offered to drive me to the doctor's office. I left the house with an ample supply of bath towels for the half-hour drive. I was soaked, and in so much pain that I didn't think I would make it through the day. When my mother stopped for gas, the attendant asked if I was in labour. I was too ill to be embarrassed.

I could tell that the gynecologist was somewhat shocked by my condition. After examining me, he said that the excessive flow of urine had caused my incision to open up; it would have to be re-sewn. He removed my urine-soaked clothes, put me in two disposable gowns, and asked my mother to drive me to the hospital, where I was admitted right away.

I remained in hospital for a week, during which time many tests were ordered. I still couldn't void properly, and the hospital staff had to use large catheters because I kept overflowing the smaller ones. I also had bladder spasms, which were uncomfortable, to say the least. My abdominal pain had become excruciating, and I started vomiting. When the results from the tests came in, I was told that my bladder was still perforated.

To this day, I don't know what really happened to me. Perhaps the surgeon who performed the emergency surgery didn't successfully repair the large puncture the gynecologist had made during the hysterectomy. Maybe the gynecologist had in fact perforated my bladder in two places. No one would tell me.

This time I was discharged from hospital with catheter in place and orders to leave it in until a third specialist could see me two weeks later. That specialist ordered countless tests. He wanted to give my bladder time to heal itself. Months later, it seemed unlikely that it would ever heal itself. The specialist finally did operate on me, but the third surgery wasn't successful either.

Help from a Caring Doctor

In the years that followed, I could not void properly because of extensive pelvic nerve damage. Urination was very painful. I had to use catheters all the time in order to empty my bladder. I only knew that I had to urinate when I felt severe pain in my kidneys. I tried every pain pill there was. Recurring infections, bladder spasms, and pain with intercourse seriously damaged my quality of life.

In 1997, I found a doctor who wanted to help me. He told me about a new experimental device called a sacral nerve root stimulator — a pacemaker for my bladder, he called it. The stimulator would override the damaged nerves, sending signals to my brain to tell me when I had to void. I thought it might be worth a try.

The proposed procedure wasn't available in my home province, so

I flew to another province in the summer of 1997 to undergo tests. During these tests, which took place over four days, electrodes were attached to my back to determine whether the stimulator would work for me. The tests were successful, and in December the stimulator was permanently implanted through further surgery.

Hormonal Havoc

As if my bladder problems weren't enough, after my surgery I began experiencing hot flashes and night sweats, as well as other menopausal symptoms. In the years that followed, it was difficult to determine which symptoms were linked to my ruptured bladder, which to the hysterectomy, and which to the hormonal therapy.

After the hysterectomy and oophorectomy, my gynecologist prescribed estrogen therapy in the form of 1.25 milligrams of Premarin daily. For four years, this dose effectively controlled the flushes and the night sweats. When a different gynecologist lowered my daily dose of ERT, claiming that it was too high, I started burning up all the time. Sex was painful because of vaginal dryness and the scar tissue in my abdomen and vagina. I also experienced brain fog and mood swings. I was particularly susceptible to mood swings if I didn't take my medication around the same time each day. I tried an Estraderm patch to deal with the symptoms, but it wasn't particularly effective. Now I am back on my original daily dose of Premarin. When EstroGel came on the market in 1999, I added that to my hormone regime, and the results have been satisfactory.

To control the pain with intercourse, I now receive regular external (through my stomach wall) and internal (vaginal) injections of medicine to numb my pelvic nerves. I still get bladder spasms from time to time, but certainly not as many as I used to before my stimulator was surgically implanted.

Epilogue

My story would have read differently had I known that the doctor who performed my hysterectomy was *not* a gynecologist, as he claimed to be. He was a family practitioner who should not have been allowed to perform a surgical procedure for which he was not trained. I never thought to question his qualifications, nor did it occur to me to get a qualified second opinion. Had I been in the care of a qualified and skilful surgeon, I feel I would not have had to endure the many complications created by the irreparable damage to my body.

Faith

❧

In 1993, I visited my gynecologist to discuss several symptoms related to my menstrual cycle. I suffered from painful menstrual cramps (dysmenorrhea) and, like many other women, premenstrual syndrome. By 1992, I had pressure-like pain in my pelvis that radiated down my thighs. My periods had become excessively heavy and were lasting longer. I missed work every month because of menstrual cramps, a fact that was duly noted on my job evaluations. My doctor said it sounded like endometriosis.

Other than those symptoms, a disc problem in my lower back, and the occasional migraine, my overall health was good and I was physically fit. At the time I consulted with the gynecologist, however, I was being treated for clinical depression. I was trying to cope with my mother's illness — she was battling breast cancer and would pass away in July of that year. I was probably not in the right frame of mind to be considering hysterectomy, especially since, as I would find out later, it can lead to or exacerbate depression in so many women.

My gynecologist ordered an ultrasound. It showed that the lining of my uterus had thickened and that I had a small cyst on my right ovary. He said that a D&C to remove the endometrium might help manage my symptoms in the short term, but that hysterectomy was the definitive treatment.

He told me that the hysterectomy would leave me virtually unchanged as a woman. The only differences would be that I would no longer have periods and their accompanying pain, and I would no longer be able to bear children. I would keep my ovaries, so I would retain hormonal function. I asked if the surgery would change my sex life. I had recently remarried and, for the first time in my life, I was enjoying sexual intimacy. I didn't want to lose that bond with my new husband. The doctor told me that sex would be even better after the operation, because I wouldn't have to worry about getting pregnant. I believed him — he made it sound so easy, so trivial, "no big deal." "We do this every day!" he said.

In the end, my decision to have the hysterectomy was based on my career. I was a registered nurse and I loved my work. After my family, my career was everything to me. I loved helping people and treating and being an advocate for my patients. But my employers were giving me a hard time about the amount of sick leave I took, and I knew that my continuing absences could hurt my chances of advancement. I didn't enjoy missing work either, and hoped that the operation would mean I could continue to do my job, only better.

My doctor suggested a laparoscopy-assisted vaginal hysterectomy, or LAVH. In this relatively new procedure, the surgeon uses an instrument called a laparoscope, which is equipped with a camera, to help visualize the pelvic cavity. The laparoscope is inserted through a tiny incision in the abdomen, and another surgical instrument to detach the uterus is inserted through a similar incision. Once the uterus has been freed from its surrounding ligaments and blood vessels, it is removed through the vagina.

It would be a simple, uncomplicated procedure, with fewer risks and less pain than abdominal surgery, said my gynecologist. I would spend less time in the hospital (three days versus the usual five) and I would enjoy a quicker recovery period, enabling me to return to my regular routine within just four weeks. LAVH was also attractive to me because my doctor could treat my endometriosis at the same time. (Ironically, my case of endometriosis was only very minor, and I now know that endometriosis is more effectively treated with abdominal surgery, so that the doctor can examine the entire pelvic cavity.)

My doctor led me to believe that hysterectomy is simply the removal of a diseased organ, like an inflamed appendix or infected tonsils. Since he made it sound so inconsequential, I agreed to undergo the procedure.

I was thirty-five years old. I should have been told much more before I consented to this procedure. But I had no reason to doubt my doctor. I thought that if there were more to tell, he would have told me. Today I know better — hysterectomy *is* a big deal.

"Call if You Have Any Problems"

The morning of the surgery, I was nervous. I couldn't tell if the butter-flies in my stomach were a normal reaction to the prospect of surgery, but my every inclination was to go back home, that this wasn't what I was supposed to be doing. My instincts told me, "I don't really need this. I need rest. There's got to be something else I can do instead of hysterectomy." However, my medical background made me feel that I would be a wimp if I changed my mind and went home. Going against my gut feeling, I stayed at the hospital and had the surgery.

After my operation, the gynecologist told me that he had accidentally hit a blood vessel with an instrument, but he had repaired it. I had been retching and vomiting all night, and I had severe abdominal pain, as well as excruciating, burning pelvic pain. Never before had I experienced so much pain, and I had given birth twice! Though it had been only a few hours since my surgery, the doctor said that I would feel better at home, and that I should call his office if there were any problems to report. He prescribed over-the-counter Tylenol for the pain.

I was discharged in the morning, just eighteen hours after the operation. By six o'clock that evening, my abdomen was quite distended. The Tylenol wasn't controlling the pain, I was still retching, and, obviously, I couldn't eat. A friend and colleague called me, and I told her about my discomfort. By then, I was feeling quite weak and dizzy, with intermittent chest pain and shortness of breath. She felt that I needed medical help, and she accompanied my husband and me when we drove to the nearest hospital.

There I was given immediate attention. The medical staff ordered oxygen, blood tests, intravenous medication for the pain and the nausea, and X-rays. My friend had a look at the X-rays with the attending physician, and she noted that part of my colon was distended — it looked as big as a football.

I was diagnosed with a bowel obstruction, known as an ileus. My intestines had temporarily stopped moving, so I couldn't pass gas or digest food. An ileus can be triggered by intense pain, manipulation of pelvic organs, foreign materials in the abdomen or pelvis, or certain medications. I was admitted for observation, rehydration, and pain management. The hospital staff were quite surprised that I had been discharged so soon after my hysterectomy. I was more surprised, however, when they said they had never heard of a procedure called LAVH!

Second Surgery

The next day I saw a general surgeon. After more tests, he determined that I had an acute abdomen, meaning that I required immediate surgery. The ultrasound showed free fluid, which meant that something had ruptured or that I was bleeding internally. The intravenous X-ray test of my kidneys and ureter showed that my right kidney was mildly distended with urine because of an obstruction of the urinary tract.

The surgeon thought that my bowel had been perforated, which was why I needed further surgery. I was feeling quite ill and very afraid, and I refused. I told the doctor that I wanted to go back to the original hospital, where everyone knew me. The surgeon, however, said that he had already spoken to the gynecologist who had performed my hysterectomy, and he convinced me that I would be fine where I was. He also pointed out that I was too sick for a hospital transfer, which would cause an unnecessary and risky delay of the surgery I needed. So I consented to a second surgery.

As it turned out, my bowel hadn't been perforated. Instead, the surgeon found multiple bleeding sites in my abdomen, with a blood clot over my right ureter, the tube that connects the kidney to the bladder. My gynecologist should never have left me with bleeding tissues after surgery. They can lead to adhesions, which, in turn, can lead to a host of medical problems. Later I was told that a gynecologist had to be called in to help the general surgeon, and they did all they could to repair the damage and stop the bleeding.

This was a far cry from what was supposed to have been a simple and uncomplicated procedure. Now I had to recover from not only vaginal surgery, but also abdominal surgery. And there would be more severe scarring because of the manipulation of my intestines and from irritation by the blood that had sat in my abdomen for almost forty-eight hours after the hysterectomy.

This time I was sent home from the hospital after seven days. Recovery was slow. I developed problems with voiding, bowel movement, and digestion. But, at my six-week checkup, neither the general surgeon nor the gynecologist appeared overly concerned about the problems I reported.

Complications

The gynecologist who performed my LAVH told me that I could slowly resume sexual activity after a couple of weeks. When my husband and I tried to be intimate, however, I felt intense pain deep inside my vagina, pain that radiated into my rectum, lower abdomen, both buttocks, and vulva and clitoral area. Now I know why. Five years after my hysterectomy, a doctor finally told me that I have a great deal of scarring at the vaginal vault (the top of the vagina, where the surgeon makes a U-shaped fold, or "cuff," after removing the cervix), and that the right and left sides are considerably different. This process also shortened my vagina, making penetrative sex even more difficult.

My problems with digestion persisted. I felt as though my intestines were blocked, and I had bladder spasms. I often felt as though I needed to urinate, only to discover that I couldn't empty my bladder completely. Mostly I dribbled, with only slight relief.

In 1994, I saw a urologist about these symptoms. He performed a cystoscopy, a procedure during which an instrument with a tiny camera is inserted into the urethra so the doctor can look at the bladder and the ureter. During this procedure, the urologist noted scarring and tears in my bladder wall. He was able to hyperdistend my bladder, but it began to bleed because it had shrunk from the scarring. He noted adhesions known as strictures in my urethra after taking a biopsy of the lining of my bladder, and explained that I have a condition called interstitial cystitis (IC), cause unknown. To manage it, the urologist told me, I would require cystoscopic procedures periodically for the rest of my life.

While the cause of my IC may have been "unknown," I knew that I didn't have any of those symptoms before the hysterectomy. I was pretty certain that my bladder troubles were linked to the LAVH.

Barely Coping

In August 1995, I underwent yet another surgery, this time to remove a small mass in my pelvis that doctors couldn't identify. During the procedure, the surgeons found severe, dense scarring which had somehow fused my intestines. Parts of them were attached to the pelvic walls and the vaginal vault, and my shrivelled left ovary was attached to my appendix. Both the ovary and my appendix were removed. After the surgery, the doctor said he had removed as many of the adhesions as possible. The mass, he said, appeared to have been caused by the bunching of my intestines.

I developed more abdominal pain. My doctor felt it was caused by impaired ovulation, resulting in painful cyst formation. I had been on Lupron, but it hadn't helped. In November 1996, my right ovary was removed. After the loss of my second ovary, my libido went from low to nil. Even with hormone replacement therapy, my sex life was far from "better than ever," as my original doctor had promised.

These later surgeries did little to alleviate the symptoms I had reported since my hysterectomy. Now that I had been castrated, I also had to contend with the many symptoms of surgical menopause: intense hot flushes, palpitations, brain fog, interrupted sleep, migraines, mood swings, loss of libido — you name it, I had it. I knew that estrogen replacement therapy could relieve me of some of those symptoms. I also knew that estrogen helps to prevent osteoporosis. Because I was susceptible to this condition, estrogen therapy had some advantages for me.

But ERT also increases a woman's risk of developing breast cancer. Given my mother's recent death from this disease, I was justifiably afraid of using estrogen. However, I do take estrogen and progesterone sporadically in cream form to help relieve my acute symptoms of surgical menopause, and also to try to stop the osteoporosis that eventually developed in my legs, hips, and lower back.

New Problems

During most of 1997, I suffered from a new pain in the right upper quadrant of my abdomen, and I continued to have little or no appetite. I was diagnosed with gallstones in 1998, another longer-term effect of hysterectomy. I was also referred to a bowel specialist. I couldn't help but wonder at the irony of it. Now there were no longer any female organs to remove or blame for my problems, doctors seemed to be more willing to investigate the vaginal pain radiating to my rectum, pelvis, and buttock.

Finally, I was diagnosed with fibromyalgia. I know very little about this disease, but I do know that its symptoms resemble those of surgical menopause. In my case, I suffer greatly from severe insomnia, impaired cognition (including poor memory and concentration), multiple joint pain, bone pain, disabling headaches, ringing in the ears, dizziness and occasional vertigo, generalized fatigue, lack of stamina, digestive problems, and pain caused by unhealthy weight loss. I also continue to suffer from hot flushes, night sweats, and loss of libido.

Wishing I Could Go Back in Time

Hindsight is 20/20. Had I known then what I know now, I can say with certainty that I would not have opted for a hysterectomy.

I later found out that the gynecologist who performed the LAVH had learned this procedure on a weekend course, where he practised on pigs. He had made it sound as though he were experienced in this complex procedure. In fact, I was the ninth woman he had performed it on — a guinea pig, one step up from his original "patients."

I had opted for hysterectomy because of my career. How ironic, then, that hysterectomy and its aftereffects cost me my job. I returned to work on modified duty just a few weeks after the LAVH. The ensuing health problems, pain, and additional surgeries, plus the onset of menopausal symptoms, caused me to miss more work than dysmenorrhea ever had. On March 16, 1998, I had to leave the hospital where I worked because of pain from gallstones. I didn't know it then, but that would be my last day of employment as a registered nurse. I am very angry about that. It's one thing to choose not to work any more; it's another to have your job taken away from you because of somebody else's lies and betrayal.

Physical pain wasn't the only thing that prevented me from doing my job the way I wanted to. In 1994, I sued the doctor who had performed my hysterectomy — a doctor who worked at the same hospital as I did. Not only did I see this man once or twice a week after my own botched surgery, but I also saw other women on whom he had performed the same operation. I would get flashbacks, and was eventually diagnosed with post-traumatic stress disorder. It became very difficult for me to stay neutral and strong for my patients.

When the lawsuit became public knowledge, as it eventually did, my colleagues — nurses and doctors who had once respected me — didn't want anything to do with me. That was very demoralizing. Physical pain is one thing, but I found it almost impossible to bear that I had lost the respect of my co-workers. I was viewed as an enemy, not a colleague; someone to be watched, not trusted. Any rapport we had built up was gone. Eventually I dropped the case. I found it impossible to find a doctor who would testify that my gynecologist hadn't met acceptable "standards of practice."

People often tell me that, as a registered nurse, I should have been more knowledgeable about the risks linked to hysterectomy. However, my training and experience were mainly in tending to the immediate needs of the ill, not in diagnosing illness or recommending treatment. That domain still belongs to physicians and surgeons.

Recently I have found a doctor — a pain management specialist — whose work I admire and whom I am slowly growing to trust. He invited me to speak at a medical information night on pelvic pain from the patient's perspective. Afterwards, most of the questions were directed at me. The experience was enormously validating. For the first time in a long time, I felt as though I were helping again. Maybe this story is another way to help.

Gayle

❦

During a routine appointment for a Pap test, my gynecologist asked me if I had any pain with intercourse. It was a question he often asked during checkups.

"No," I said, "no problem there, but I have been having really bad, knife-sharp pains with bowel movements."

I was a little hesitant to tell him about these pains. After all, bowel problems weren't really his area. He addressed my complaint, however, and did a rectal exam. When he said that he felt "something in there," I was immediately concerned. The gynecologist's best guess was that I had endometriosis. After some thought, he decided to schedule me for laparoscopic surgery to investigate the cause of my pain.

When my gynecologist told me that this procedure was the only definitive way to diagnose endometriosis, I readily agreed. Because I was complaining of heavy periods and we knew I had a small fibroid tumour in my uterus, he said that he would also do a hysteroscopy (an examination of the uterine cavity using an instrument called a hysteroscope, which is inserted through the vagina and cervix) and a D&C to scrape away the endometrial tissue and relieve — at least temporarily — my heavy periods.

Although I worried that these exploratory surgeries might turn up evidence of disease, I was also happy that I might finally have some answers about — and perhaps relief from — the mysterious medical problems that had plagued me for so long. I had noticed that many of my symptoms seemed cyclical and related to menstruation, and had been thinking what a relief it would be to reach menopause, when I wouldn't have to contend with those problems any more.

I had been struggling for years with extremely heavy, clotted periods. When I mentioned this problem to my gynecologist during a routine appointment, he told me it was a normal occurrence. "As you age, your period can become heavy and you can get lots of clots." As well, I had suffered for years from diarrhea at menstruation, and I began to bleed rectally during my periods, which alarmed me.

I also had strange pains that I couldn't explain. I had been prescribed anti-inflammatory drugs countless times for inflammations that would flare up over and over again in various limbs. In the years leading up to this particular doctor's visit, I had had numerous X-rays to diagnose the source of the pain and a cortisone injection in my thigh to help control the inflammation.

Sinus congestion had become a monthly occurrence; it felt as though someone were driving a nail into my right temple. And during each cycle, I experienced sharp, needle-like pains in my urethra and a pain under my ribcage that I found difficult to explain to the doctor. The worst pains came after my period ended, when my abdomen was so bloated and sore it often hurt just to sit down.

My family doctor had never suggested that endometriosis might be the cause of all these various problems. He had grown accustomed to hearing me describe strange pains that came and went, and I often wondered if he thought of me as a hypochondriac, the way my husband did. I was even beginning to think that way myself. But my problems were all too *real* to be imaginary. I couldn't understand why new symptoms kept cropping up, and why doctors couldn't explain their cause.

When I began having terrible pain with bowel movements, however, I knew I couldn't ignore them, so I decided to discuss them with my doctor. As fate would have it, I was scheduled for a Pap test with my gynecologist before I would see my general practitioner again. And that was how I found myself scheduled for exploratory surgery.

"I Might Do a Hysterectomy"

In the two weeks leading up to my surgery, I worried about what the doctor might find — cancer? At the same time, I hoped that the D&C would bring some relief from my heavy periods. I was also anxious to learn what was causing my bowel problems. The doctor had given me a short pamphlet about endometriosis. After I read it, I still didn't feel I knew much about the disease. It did say that endometrial tissue could grow on the bowel and cause problems, and I wondered if this was what had happened in my case. Well, I thought, there would be time for all my questions after the exploratory surgery.

In the hospital on the day of my operation, I was already scrubbed and prepped for surgery when the gynecologist arrived. He briefly discussed the procedures, adding that if he found lots of endometrial implants in my abdomen, he might do a hysterectomy at the same time. I remember how casually he made that suggestion, without discussing the possible ramifications of the procedure. I agreed, just as casually, that removing my uterus would be a good idea.

The gynecologist seemed reluctant to ask his next question, "What about your ovaries?" He seemed to be mulling over my options and his recommendation. Finally he said that if I had only a mild case of endometriosis, he would leave my ovaries intact. If he found a severe case, the decision was an easy one — he would remove them.

"What would you like me to do with your ovaries if the endometriosis is only moderate?" he asked.

I knew little about the importance of the ovaries, other than that they produced estrogen. But the idea of losing them gave me pause. I wondered how I might feel without any female organs. Would I feel less of a woman? Would there be side effects beyond the end of my periods and long-awaited relief from my strange pains and health problems? I thought of my three healthy children, and how much I had enjoyed being pregnant and giving birth. But I wasn't planning on having any more children. My youngest was thirteen at the time, and I honestly thought I didn't really need my ovaries any more.

"Take them out," I said. "I won't be needing them anyway. I don't want to wake up only to find out that I need another surgery."

The doctor still seemed hesitant, as if there were more he wished to tell me. There was so little time for discussion of any kind. I wish he had talked to me about the potential risks and side effects of hysterectomy and removal of the ovaries and cervix. I wish he had told me of the effects those surgeries could have on my sex life. Had he mentioned any of those things to me, I know I would have asked him to hold off on the hysterectomy and oophorectomy until I could do the research. However, he didn't say anything more. I was wheeled into the operating room and was soon unconscious under the anesthetic.

Hysterectomized and Forgotten

When I came out of the anesthesia, I learned that the doctor had performed a total abdominal hysterectomy and bilateral salpingo-oophorectomy. During the operation he had sent word to my husband that my right ovary was adhered to my uterus, and that he would be removing all of my reproductive organs.

I was anxious to discuss my surgery with the doctor. Unfortunately, I didn't get to talk to him until two weeks had passed. Apparently he had gone on holiday immediately following my hysterectomy and had obviously forgotten all about me. I was upset enough when I learned the extent of my surgery, but I was even more troubled when I found that the doctor wasn't available to explain exactly why he had gone ahead with the total hysterectomy.

The day after my hysterectomy, a nurse brought me a hormone patch. She explained that the doctor had prescribed it for me, and that I should put it on right away. But I understood that endometriosis was stimulated by estrogen. Wouldn't taking estrogen right away lead to more problems? The nurse couldn't answer any of my questions, so I refused to put on the patch.

Let the Healing Begin

In the weeks that followed, I tried to concentrate on healing. My external scars — a six-inch abdominal incision and the tiny laparoscopic incision above it — healed quickly. Adjusting to the extensive internal changes that surgery had made to my anatomy would take longer. My husband and teenage children were busy with their own lives and activities, so I was grateful for my parents' help. For the most part I handled my business activities by phone, and some other things just didn't get done.

As I had time to spare during my recovery, I started reading about hysterectomy and hormone replacement therapy. My sister sent me two books, *What Your Doctor May Not Tell You About Menopause*, by Dr. John Lee, and *Estrogen*, by Dr. Lila Anchtigall and Joan Heilman. Once I was able to go out, I bought various other books on endometriosis and hysterectomy, and soon realized how little has been written for women like me. I read that endometriosis could come back even without the use of replacement hormones, and that taking hormone replacements could greatly increase this risk. And much to my dismay, I read that women should retain their uteruses and ovaries at all costs, except in the case of cancer.

The Aftereffects

Immediately after surgery, I began to experience hot flashes and night sweats. I got little sleep during my first few weeks home from the hospital. At night I would awaken, drenched with sweat. In the daytime, I was overcome by heat and a panicky, "let-me-out-of-this-skin" feeling. It was bad, but I told myself I could live with it, provided I didn't suffer other symptoms. I stood firm against hormone replacement therapy, and eventually the hot flashes bothered me less. Over time, they became so infrequent and slight that I can honestly say they were the very least of my problems.

In spite of my decreased libido, I was eager to resume sexual activity with my husband. I wanted to be reassured that our sexual intimacy would continue as it had been before my surgery. In the first few months, intercourse was painful and difficult, and I ached for hours afterward. I was unhappily surprised to discover that my post-surgery orgasms paled in comparison with what they had been before the hysterectomy. Instead of ocean waves of response, there were shallow ripples. I soon realized from my reading on the subject that this effect was permanent — nothing would ever bring back the intense and highly pleasurable orgasms that come from a contracting uterus and stimulated cervix. I felt as though a great gift had been taken away from me.

Over time, my vaginal dryness increased to the point where penetration made me bleed. I saw another gynecologist, and readily accepted his prescription for estrogen in cream form, hoping it would resolve my problem. Two weeks after I started using the cream, however, I suffered from vaginal soreness and irritation, and had to stop the treatment. I wondered when I would be as good as new again, and when my libido and vaginal secretions would return.

I reported back to the gynecologist who had performed my hysterectomy. He diagnosed a yeast infection and persuaded me to try the hormone patch. I worried about the possible side effects of the patch. In particular, I was concerned about the possibility of blood clots, as I had experienced years earlier. I wore the patch for exactly ten days, until

I woke up one night with intense, knife-like pains in my chest. My doctor agreed that I should no longer use the patch, and recommended that I try the estrogen cream again. I did, but once again developed a troublesome yeast infection. Would there ever be an end to this?

I have since tried all the moisturizing vaginal creams, without success. I have also visited several different gynecologists; none of them gave me more than a cursory exam and all of them had one standard answer — hormone replacement therapy in the form of a pill or patch. When I questioned one doctor about the possibility of using herbs or supplements to increase my libido, he told me, rather snidely, "When the engine's gone, no amount of gas is going to get it going again." I felt terrible when I left his office!

My already diminished libido gradually disappeared altogether. What did not disappear, however, was my desire for the closeness and intimacy that sexual intercourse brought to my marriage. My difficulties in having normal sexual intercourse strained our relationship. As a normal sex life and any semblance of desire on my part became things of the past, I grieved most of all for the loss to my marriage. Sexual intimacy had always been a bond that brought my husband and me together. Those times of closeness were especially important after we had disagreed or fought. Because my husband is not naturally an affectionate person, the touching and holding that come with the sex act were especially valuable to me.

My husband found it extremely hard to discuss his feelings about the changes my hysterectomy had created. I pressed him to express how he felt, and he finally admitted that he was very bitter, accusing me of undergoing the hysterectomy to avoid sex. I was heartsick, and so depressed. At the very time when I needed comfort and reassurance, I was being chastised. Our sex life continued, but achieving orgasm became strained and tedious. The joy now seems to have gone out of intimacy, and my husband, still hurt by what he perceives as my wilful disregard for his happiness, rarely initiates sex. We have been married for twenty-one years. Our marriage, like most, has been filled with struggles. Ironically, I felt that we would always have great sex to carry us through the problems. Now that outlet is gone, and the relationship has been dealt a huge blow.

If my husband found it difficult to understand the vast physiological changes wrought by the removal of major, hormone-producing organs, it also took me years to realize the full extent of the loss I had suffered and to attempt to come to terms with it. Other health issues surfaced in the months following my hysterectomy. I noticed a change in the texture of my hair and the resiliency of my skin; both seemed dry and lifeless. But I tell myself that I can handle "cosmetic" changes more easily than those that suggest my physical and emotional health and well-being have been compromised.

I have substantially less energy and stamina. My bones are thinning; when my mother informed me that she had been diagnosed with osteoporosis, I immediately began taking Fosamax to prevent the disease. I have been diagnosed with rosacea, a skin disease that causes redness and acne flare-ups on the face. I have irritable bowel syndrome, my cholesterol has risen to unacceptable levels, and my eyes show early signs of macular degeneration.

All of these unpleasant developments took place in the year following my surgery. I immediately suspected that they were all related to the hysterectomy. Although I was relieved to have an end to the mysterious inflammations throughout my body and the sharp pain and heavy blood loss of periods, suddenly I was faced with yet more daunting problems. No one had warned me.

When I read stories about women who had hysterectomies in their twenties, I think how lucky I was to have had my uterus, ovaries, and other reproductive organs for forty-eight years, and to have had three wonderful children as a result. Some women have suffered far more than I have. But sometimes, when I'm struck by the negative impacts of hysterectomy on my life, all I can do is cry.

I continue to try to find ways to regain the quality of life I had before my hysterectomy. My efforts have been both frustrating and depressing.

Recently I found a female gynecologist who has prescribed vaginal estrogen in the form of a pill. I have been able to tolerate this treatment, which has been helpful in healing my vaginal tissue to some extent, and has given me some hope for the future. In the meantime, my journey to better health continues.

I feel a great underlying sadness when I think of the many changes in my life that followed my surgery, and the impact it has had on my marriage. Looking back, I think of the day I had my hysterectomy — even though I had just turned forty-eight — as the day I got old.

Eve

❧

About a year and a half after my hysterectomy, I made one of my many trips to the pharmacy to pick up a refill of "don't-pee-your-pants" medicine. As I pulled into a parking space, I saw a flashy red sports car parked directly in front of mine. A well-dressed middle-aged man strode confidently towards the car, carrying his purchases. His demeanour suggested that — as my nineteen-year-old son might say — he had the world by the 'nads. My hands began to tremble as I suddenly realized that this man did indeed have the world by the gonads — mine, and those of the numerous other women who had paid for that shiny red car with our blood and our tears and our precious reproductive organs. This man was none other than the proud proprietor of our local "Hysterectomies-R-Us" establishment.

As I sat, shaking, in my car, I began to relive, in fragmented memories and painful flashbacks, my unnecessary hysterectomy gone painfully wrong. I remembered vividly the many colours of urine: urine so contaminated with blood that it was a deep, dark burgundy; urine dyed the orange colour of a school bus by a medicine called peridium; urine the colour of indigo because my bladder was so scarred that doctors had to use dye to determine if a stent could be inserted through it or through my kidney. I remembered vomiting a greenish-yellow liquid and thinking that it too was urine. (I later learned from my urologist that it was bile.)

I also remembered voices and apologies:

"I'm so sorry, but I didn't do this. My partner did."

"I'm sorry, the surgery to remove the stitch that is creating the blockage in your ureter was unsuccessful. I was also unable to get the stent in because of inflammation and swelling."

"I'm sorry, the surgery to insert the stent through your bladder was unsuccessful."

"Just look at all the adhesions in her bladder!"

"You'll have to take this medicine for the rest of your life."

"There's a chance your ureter could close up again."

"You've been through hell."

One voice stood out in particular — the essence of pain. Some poor woman was screaming and making guttural, tortured sounds from deep within her soul as a stent was inserted directly into her kidney without anesthesia. It scraped the inside of her bladder, already raw, swollen, and inflamed from a botched "repair" job. I had never in my life heard such primal screams of pain, and I hope never to hear them again. I remembered the emotions that flooded through me when I recognized that tormented voice — it was my own.

Lies, Lies and More Lies

As the man tossed his bag into his car, I looked at his mouth and remembered some of the many lies that had poured from it:

"If you don't have a hysterectomy, your uterus is going to fall right through your vagina."

"You'll feel so much better."

"The testosterone in the hormone supplement I'm giving you will make you horny."

"This happened because you have an abnormal arc to your pubic bone."

"Your bladder won't be nicked during the hysterectomy."

"If your bladder is damaged, of course your urologist will be the one to repair it."

"This happened because of the urology surgeons who operated before."

Lies, lies, and more lies. Lies in my medical chart that said I was advised that a compromised ureter and urinary incontinence were "acceptable risks." Lies designed to make a woman believe that sex would improve after a hysterectomy.

The Indignation of it all

I remembered humiliation and indignity. I remembered a nurse teaching my husband how to empty my two catheters and how to take care of the dressing at the site of my nephrostomy tube, which was inserted directly into my kidney so I could empty my bladder despite my blocked ureter. I was standing there in a hospital gown with my backside exposed as another hospital employee walked in. I remembered how I felt when my husband had to teach my son how to empty my catheters. I remembered wetting myself at a grocery store. I remembered the times when I had to wake my husband in the middle of the night because I had wet the bed or my nephrostomy tube had sprung a leak. I remembered lying with my legs in stirrups during a cystoscopy as two doctors and a nurse examined the adhesions in my bladder, as if I were nothing more than a scarred organ to them. I remembered running into an acquaintance at the store with nothing in my shopping cart except Poise pads and rectal suppositories, which have also become a fact of my life since the hysterectomy.

As the man started up the motor of his shiny red car, I sat and thought about frustration. I remembered how much it hurt to see the look on my husband's face after our pathetic attempts at sex. A faint smile appeared briefly on my face as I thought for a few seconds about our fulfilling sex life before the hysterectomy. A flash of despair quickly replaced the smile as I thought about how a former source of pleasure had been replaced by strife, contention, and frustration. I remembered looking into my husband's blue eyes and seeing the inadequacy he felt — he had somehow failed to protect me, and now he could no more invoke sexual arousal in me than in an inanimate object. I thought about him knocking softly on the bathroom door after we tried to make love, apologizing for hurting me as he listened to my wrenching, uncontrollable sobs on the other side of the door.

New Realities

I remembered the frustration I felt when I returned to work and couldn't follow the discussions at meetings. I had completely lost my ability to concentrate. Before my hysterectomy, I ran the meetings at work. After the surgery, I merely attended them, only pretending to understand the issues on the agenda.

As the man in the car looked over his shoulder to back out, I was confronted with the fears that have become part of my everyday existence. I am afraid that I will lose my job; because of my severe lack of energy, my inability to concentrate, and short-term memory loss, I can no longer pull my weight at work. I used to be friendly, vibrant, and focused — a mover and a shaker. Now I am just the pitiful, lonely soul who sits in her cubicle all day, speaking to no one unless spoken to. I eat my lunch alone at my desk since the hysterectomy.

I am also afraid my husband will someday leave me. He is a handsome, virile man; when acquaintances see us together I can read their minds as they wonder what he could possibly see in his overweight drudge of a wife. *She's really let herself go in the past few years.*

As the man in the flashy red car backed out of his parking spot, our eyes met briefly. I searched his for a flicker of recognition. I saw none. For a moment I was overwhelmed and enraged with the certain knowledge that he didn't even recognize me. I was absolutely nothing to him. In perhaps two short hours, however, he had ruined almost every aspect of my life and completely destroyed so much of what was important to me.

Then I caught a glance at myself in the rear-view mirror and realized why the man in the red car didn't recognize me. I no longer even slightly resembled the happy, healthy, attractive, vibrant woman who had been wheeled into the operating room that cold February morning.

As the shiny red car backed out of its parking space, I reached for my purse. I was about to get out of my car when I hesitated. I gazed again at the red car and remembered something else important. I suddenly knew there was something I just had to do.

I remembered the many, many nights I had gone to bed at night wishing I would never again awake, only to get up each morning to the nightmare that was now my life. I bowed my head and prayed a silent, fervent prayer for the next happy, healthy, attractive, vibrant woman whose destiny it was to be wheeled into that man's operating room.

As I finished my prayer, it suddenly occurred to me that I did, in fact, have one body part that still functioned normally. I raised my right hand, palm towards me, and extended my middle finger at the shiny red car as it drove out of sight.

Roberta

❧

In 1992, during my yearly Pap test, a nurse practitioner found a fibroid tumour on the back wall of my uterus. That discovery began what would be a seven-year struggle to hang on to my reproductive organs.

There had been heavier bleeding with my periods in recent years, but since I had suffered with PMS all my life, it was just one more inconvenience. I had no symptoms that I associated with something more serious. I had never even heard of fibroids.

My initial reaction, beyond worry, was to read up on fibroids. When I discovered hysterectomy was the standard method for dealing with them, I read up on that as well.

Books I read reported that there were no problems associated with a hysterectomy. Doctors who performed the surgical procedure repeatedly stated that the only purpose that the uterus served was for reproduction, and once a woman was finished having children she was better off without it. They reported that most women were happy to be rid of their monthly periods, however, there were several books, also written by doctors, which spoke of how a hysterectomy had the potential to affect a woman's health and quality of life. These doctors maintained that there were alternatives to hysterectomy, such as a myomectomy, to deal with fibroids. A myomectomy was a procedure where only the fibroids were removed leaving the woman's uterus and other parts of her reproductive system intact, thus protecting her health.

A hysterectomy was a frightening thought for me although I didn't know why. I had no plans to have children, but still there was an instinctive fear of losing my uterus. Removing it I felt could create problems for me in ways that I didn't yet know.

Fighting to Keep my Uterus

Armed with the knowledge I was acquiring from books, I told the first gynecologist I saw about some of the problems associated with a hysterectomy, and I asked her about having a myomectomy to get rid of my fibroids. My information about post hysterectomy problems was brushed off. I was advised that with a myomectomy fibroids grow back. She told me that if I were to get married tomorrow, and my husband really wanted children, she would try to save my uterus. Otherwise it had to come out. She added that the cervix and the ovaries would need to be removed at the same time to prevent the possibility of developing cancer some time in the future.

I couldn't understand why my uterus only had value if a man was attached to it. After all, I was attached to it in more ways than one. I also couldn't understand why healthy body parts like my ovaries and cervix needed to be removed to prevent the possibility of cancer in the future. But she was insistent and refused to listen to my pleas to keep my uterus and other parts of my reproductive system.

I still couldn't envision having a hysterectomy, especially not for a fibroid, a condition that is most often benign. And certainly not in light of the information I was gathering on hysterectomies. I held out hope that I would find a gynecologist who would be sympathetic to my desire to keep my uterus.

A year later, the next gynecologist I saw threatened to show me a kidney dialysis unit if I didn't have a hysterectomy. She told me that was where I was going to end up because the fibroid could grow to the point where it pressed on the kidneys, damaging them. Like the first gynecologist, she too insisted that the cervix and the ovaries had to come out to prevent the possibility of developing cancer in the future. She also denied there were any problems associated with a hysterectomy even when I brought up specific examples. I asked her if she knew of a doctor who did myomectomies. Although she worked in a clinic and at a hospital with other gynecologists, and her husband was a gynecologist, she said she did not. She made no offer to try and find a doctor who did.

I continued to resist the pressure from gynecologists and family practitioners to have a hysterectomy, and kept on with my research. Friends didn't understand my refusal either. They had known many women who had undergone this common surgical procedure and had been very happy with it. Some claimed it was the best thing they'd ever done, and that they wished they had done it sooner. All of this pressure, combined with a uterus that was growing in size to where it had expanded my abdomen to the size of a six-month pregnancy, exerted enormous stress on me. Clothes didn't fit anymore, tying a shoe meant unzipping my pants, sleeping on my stomach was difficult and some people asked me if I was pregnant.

Finally, a new family doctor showed some empathy, and offered to help me find a surgeon who did less radical procedures for fibroids. I agreed to go for an appointment with the gynecologist she recommended, hoping against hope that he would be willing to save my uterus. In his opinion, however, the fibroids had grown too large to perform a myomectomy but, after some pleading from me, he was agreeable to leaving my cervix and ovaries behind.

Giving in and Hoping for the Best

It seemed that there were no other options left. I was desperate and exhausted with what had become a seven-year struggle to keep my uterus. Hoping that all my research and gut feelings were wrong and the doctors were right, I gave in and I had a hysterectomy. I awoke to find out that my cervix had been left in, but only one ovary. A cyst had been discovered on the other one, and the entire ovary had been removed. My family doctor agrees with me that the surgeon could have used a laser to remove just the cyst, saving that ovary.

Initially, my recovery was very good. I was so happy with my new-found energy, a flat stomach and clothes that I could now fit into. I could even bend down to tie my shoes with no difficulty. I was determined to maintain a positive attitude about the hysterectomy in the hope that it would translate into a good outcome with none of the complications I had read about in my research.

On my first day home from the hospital, I experienced painful cramping and diarrhea every time I ate, occasionally vomiting as well. I knew I didn't have this problem before the surgery. Sometimes it took just one bite of a sandwich to send me to the bathroom in excruciating pain much worse than any menstrual cramps I had ever had. It became impossible to leave the house for a couple of hours after consuming food of any kind. Going to work became difficult if I ate. When I was out with friends one evening at a restaurant, I spent two hours in the washroom with vomiting, diarrhea and cramps while my friends finished dinner. After that I realized I could no longer socialize if it involved food. Travelling became impossible, because I needed a bathroom close at hand at all times!

It was only after many difficult months of pain that I learned that estrogen plays a significant role in the digestive system, and that my problem was related to the drop in estrogen levels in my body following the hysterectomy. It took nearly two years of experimenting with stool softeners and different estrogen therapies before I was able to find some relief from this irritable bowel syndrome. To this day, I still suffer from urge incontinent bowels, and I must be careful to stay close to a washroom, especially in the mornings. This problem continues to restrict my activities at certain times of the day.

Forever Changed

Within months of the surgery, I could feel a growing depression settling over me. I knew from my research that, in situations like this, that doctors often misdiagnose the problem as psychological and tend to prescribe antidepressants instead of estrogen, which is what is really needed to counter declining levels of that hormone. So, when my gynecologist offered to prescribe the antidepressant Celexa, I asked for estrogen. Thankfully, my family doctor was more willing to listen and allow me to participate in my own health care, and she prescribed the estrogen I needed. The depression lifted within days.

By this time, I knew I had to expand my education from hysterectomies and fibroids to the subject of hormones and hormone therapy. I needed to know how to treat the impact the hysterectomy had on my hormone system.

Fatigue became a growing problem. It was a strange kind of fatigue, and definitely different from anything I had ever experienced. Going to bed or sitting in a chair to rest never seemed to help. No matter how much I wanted to do things around the house, engage in some favourite activity, or even read a book, I was too wiped out to do it.

As well, my job was a very physical one, and soon I noticed that I was losing my muscle strength and stamina. Often I had to enlist the help of someone to complete my work. Around this time I was offered a full time job, but had to turn it down because the fatigue was so intense I could no longer last an entire day. One reason I had finally given in to the surgery was that I had hoped that getting rid of the fibroids would give me the energy and health I needed to return to full time employment. Heavy bleeding from the fibroids had caused anemia and fatigue. This meant that I was only able to work part time. The iron pills that were prescribed prior to the surgery brought my energy levels back to normal, and I wish now that I had stayed with that approach instead of the hysterectomy.

Having read Dr. Susan Rako's book on testosterone, I was certain that it was not depression that was causing the fatigue, despite what my doctor said. I asked her for testosterone. There is no set dose for women, so it required much experimenting to find a dose that worked for me most of the time. Although it has not returned my energy levels to the way they were before the hysterectomy, it has given me enough of my strength and energy back to be able to continue working part time.

By the third month post-operatively, I began having difficulty thinking clearly, making decisions or planning anything. My brain felt like it was full of cotton balls rather than brain cells. Tasks requiring concentration or memory became increasingly difficult to perform. Writing, something I had always loved to do, became more challenging for me. When I do write, my thoughts are often fragmented or incomplete. This erosion of my mental faculties has resulted in a decline in my self-confidence. Participating in a group discussion is something I shy away from now, as I am unable to keep up with the conversation. I seem to have tremendous difficulty retrieving information stored in my brain, which makes effective communication a problem.

Despite being on hormone therapy now, there is still a long list of problems with which I struggle to cope. Stress incontinence with my bladder, fatigue, depression, itchy skin, sleep apnea, hair loss, dental problems, personality changes and memory problems are some of the challenges I face. I know I had none of these before my hysterectomy! Apart from the fibroids and the problems they caused, my health had been good.

A leaky bladder, especially when I sneeze or cough, means I must wear bulky pads for protection. Much of the long blonde hair I had, and I liked so much, has fallen out. I am now faced with the likelihood that it will have to be cut short to disguise this considerable loss. I have developed sleep apnea where I stop breathing briefly, and wake up gasping for air. It often makes falling asleep difficult, and puts a strain on my heart.

I had always had a very good sex drive with strong orgasms. So when I noticed the decline, that the orgasms were not as strong and that it was taking me so much longer to get aroused, I knew that my sexuality had been affected by the hysterectomy and the resulting hormonal changes. Eventually most of the sensation in my pelvic region was lost, and although I fought to keep my cervix, so that there would be sexual sensation during intercourse, it is now numb. In spite of the addition of hormone therapy my sex drive has not returned to what it was previously. The actors Richard Gere and Pierce Brosnan used to look so good to me. Now I feel nothing for them or any man. I have lost the connection to my feminine side, and I no longer feel like a woman. Instead, I feel de-sexed and neutered, when it comes to my sexual identity and feelings. Before this surgery, I had repeatedly asked the doctors about the possibility of a hysterectomy affecting a woman's sex drive. All three gynecologists denied it could be affected.

High Price to Pay

Still, of all the problems that have developed as a result of my hysterectomy, the most devastating has been the impact on my personality and emotions.

From the first day home from the hospital, I noticed a lack of connection to close friends and people I have known for years and cared for a great deal. It is a terrible experience to not be able to feel love for someone you know meant the world to you. All I have now is the memory of having felt that way at one time. Gradually my emotions became flat and dull. I found myself unable to feel love, joy, sadness, and excitement or to experience any emotion intensely. This is particularly noticeable when something joyful or very sad happens. Lacking the ability to shed more than a few tears now, I haven't had a long deep cry since this happened to me. Yet I have so much more to cry about now.

I wasn't this way before my hysterectomy. I don't fully understand what has happened to me except that hormones affect the part of the brain that is involved with emotions. I realize now that this was what I had intuitively feared when I was first presented with having a hysterectomy years ago, that I would lose me. It was why I resisted it for so long. I have lost much of what it means to be human, the ability to feel emotions and to feel connected to those around me.

Through all of this, I have learned amazing things about my female body, its reproductive system and hormones. I am in awe of the complexity of this creation. Because of me, my family doctor has learned a great deal about the problems a hysterectomy can cause. She is even more hesitant now than she was when I first met her to recommend a hysterectomy for conditions where there is no cancer involved. As well, she is getting an education in hormone therapy for the hysterectomized woman, and how difficult it can be to find something that works. Although we still have not found any hormone therapy that has returned me to the way I was before this surgery, together we continue to search for a hormone therapy that will. I have begun to work to help keep other women from going through a similar experience. I have assisted in organizing educational forums in my local community on this issue for women and their health care providers. In addition, I have managed to help several women find doctors who were willing to do less radical procedures for their fibroids and endometriosis.

Of course now I realize that my body had its own inner wisdom, and that the gut feelings I had before the hysterectomy were my body's way of trying to tell me something. I wish I had trusted my instincts before so much of me was taken away.

LaShonda

❦

When I was almost forty years old, I began to suffer from hot flashes, vaginal dryness, and erratic mood swings that I believe started shortly after I had a tubal ligation. So I booked an appointment with a gynecologist thinking that a pelvic exam would help me get to the root of my problems. I was also thinking that a prescription for hormone therapy might provide me with some relief from the perimenopausal symptoms I felt were cramping my lifestyle.

Only One Option

Following my exam, the gynecologist told me that he felt several masses, including one on my left ovary. He said that my uterus was enlarged with tumours, most likely fibroids, and he added that although these growths were not yet cancerous, they soon would be and pain would follow. According to the doctor, the risk of a hemorrhage was imminent, and my only option was to undergo a hysterectomy and oophorectomy as soon as possible. And then almost as if he were talking to himself, he said he would have to do an abdominal procedure.

I was numb and confused about the news of my diseased organs. Noticing my shock, the doctor suggested that I allow myself some time to think about it.

It was hard not to think about anything else, and in the days that followed, my numbness gave way to panic. I was worried about what would become of me, and how it would affect my husband and my children. And I kept thinking I was too young to die!

Since the gynecologist recommended that I seek a second opinion from a colleague whose opinion he valued, my husband and I thought it should be our first step. Sadly, the second specialist concurred with the first one's findings, and in doing so, sealed my fate.

My gynecologist told me very little about the surgery except that my incision would be barely noticeable. He mentioned the short hospital stay, after which I would be fully recovered in a matter of weeks. He said I would need to rest and refrain from sexual activity during my recovery period, and handed me some written instructions on personal hygiene following surgery. I understood that he would prescribe hormones to help me feel much better pending the results of the pathology report. As for my sex life, he said that the hysterectomy would improve it. I should have told him that it didn't need improving.

Struggling to control my misgivings about the surgery, I entered the operating room thinking I was doing what was right for my loved ones. The room went cold and dark, and all I could hear were the surgeon's assurances that everything would be alright.

Sex Would Have to Wait

Recovery was slow, but I managed. At my post-operative visit, the doctor said that the results of the pathology report were good and I could begin taking hormones. I was grateful as the hot flashes had been horrendous up to that point. Then he explained that my incision was not healing well internally and sex would have to wait. Though my husband and I were a bit disappointed at this news, we were relieved to learn that I was cancer-free.

When our celibacy period was finally over, I noted the lack of response on my part. Sex had become uncomfortable, I felt the loss of sensation in my genitals, and of greater concern was my loss of libido. I started telling myself that it was only a matter of needing more or a different type of hormone replacement therapy (HRT).

Six months later, I went back to my gynecologist to report that I was still bleeding and that I had begun experiencing incontinence. After he examined me, he told me that the incision was likely the cause of my bleeding problem, because it was still healing. Then he said I couldn't possibly be leaking urine. His attitude toward me became cool, and although I found it odd and intimidating, I decided to talk to him about my sexual dysfunction. He dismissed that problem as something he'd never heard of before. The issue was dropped and he handed me a prescription for a different form of HRT.

I Would Never be the Same Again

I left his office in utter shock, but it was then that I decided to research hysterectomy and castration. I needed to understand what was happening to me. I researched medical textbooks at every opportunity to familiarize myself with the role of a woman's reproductive organs. Many books and studies confirmed that the ovaries, uterus and cervix play a very significant role in a woman's sexual response, in addition to making important contributions to the endocrine system (group of hormone producing organs in our body). It was becoming quite clear to me that once you remove some of the organs from the equation, the loss is felt in a variety of ways. I concluded that my sexuality would never be the same again.

What a blow! Certainly, I had never signed up for this. My femininity and my sexuality had always been an important part of me and I never wanted these to be taken away. What I wanted was to keep on being my husband's pretty and sexy wife. Prior to my hysterectomy, we'd been married over two decades and we still played games and flirted with one another. Now the games were over and the relationship strained. Once eager for his touch, I was now avoiding it. We rarely kissed and sex became a ritual to be over and done with very quickly. Afterwards, all I wanted was to be left alone so I could cry.

While I knew the estrangement troubled my husband, I found I was unable to respond emotionally. This detachment extended to my children, and later while researching more medical literature, I learned that this was a direct result of my castration. The literature showed that ovaries secrete oxytocin, the hormone of mating and maternal behaviours, and I no longer had ovaries.

I was becoming more and more fatigued. My breasts were shrinking yet I was gaining weight everywhere else. I once loved to laugh, but I could no longer find anything amusing. I felt alienated and powerless to do anything about it. Since my emotional state wasn't improving, I was thinking that perhaps my new hrt prescription wasn't helping and that I would need to look into it.

I couldn't go on pretending about what was happening between my husband and I, and eventually we talked. He admitted to feeling hurt by my inability to respond to him sexually and he too wanted the woman I was before the hysterectomy. Our discussions haven't necessarily made it any easier for us, but they have helped us to reconnect.

The Ultimate Betrayal

Later when I requested a copy of my surgical and pathology reports from the hospital, I was dealt another blow — my hysterectomy and castration had been completely unnecessary. There was no evidence of the cancerous condition that the two specialists had spoken of. Even more shocking were the results of my pre-operative tests — all were normal. I couldn't help but feel angry and betrayed.

I don't know how to overcome the anger and the betrayal knowing that my quality of life may never be the same. I continue to feel deeply saddened by the tremendous impact that this surgery has had on my sexuality and my relationship with my husband. We shared a closeness that made us look forward to each day, and we never thought it would be taken away by a surgeon's scalpel. If a woman is not warned about the threat to her sexuality prior to a hysterectomy and oophorectomy, how can it be informed consent?

Penny

❧

"You have no other choice!" That's how the hysterectomy option was presented to me. For years, I suffered from repeated bladder infections, heavy periods, pelvic pain and anemia. Maybe my doctor had a point, but I never considered hysterectomy as my only option. In fact, I was willing to try anything else.

A couple of years prior to my hysterectomy decision, I had under-gone a laparoscopy, which revealed the presence of endometriosis, but the subsequent treatments had not provided me with any relief. Although I didn't want to proceed with drastic surgery, I was looking to help myself to a better existence. I could no longer work, nor could I take adequate care of my five children. I was sick all the time, and tired of feeling that way. I started thinking that my family deserved better, and so I put my trust in my doctor.

"You'll Regret not Having it Done Earlier!"

One thing I remember my doctor telling me about hysterectomy is that it would make me feel so good, I would regret not having it done earlier. He didn't talk to me about the risks of the procedure itself or any of the potential side effects that can result from the removal of a woman's uterus. Therefore, mine was not a decision based on informed consent. But even if he had warned me of at least some of the many dangers associated with this surgery, it would have done little to prepare me for the long term and life-changing difficulties I would face.

A Difficult Recovery

I had a vaginal hysterectomy that left me unable to void. You can imagine my discomfort and my fear. While in hospital, nurses showed me how to apply a catheter to help me pass urine. They explained that this was but a temporary situation that would take care of itself once the swelling from the surgery would go down. However, this problem persisted for another 13 months, and it had a tremendous impact on my daily living.

During my first week of recovery, I started experiencing severe pain in my breasts. Though this condition is an indication of lack of estrogen in the body, my doctor dismissed the problem as imaginary. As I am not in the habit of inventing health problems, I felt slighted by his reaction to my complaint, but I let it go thinking there wouldn't be any point in alienating him. In his view, I was well and ready to resume my normal daily activities. But it's not how I felt.

A week later, I was back in his office to report a protrusion extending outward from my vagina. It was a huge bulge that had me feeling sick with worry. It occurred to me that up to this point, the hysterectomy had not made me feel very good at all. The doctor explained that my vagina had been weakened by the surgery, and that its outward protrusion was caused by pressure coming from the rectal area. If I felt shock and dismay at what was happening to me, it was nothing compared to the tremor I felt when he said that further surgery wouldn't help, and that I could learn to live with the problem. I couldn't believe what I was hearing, and I went home feeling devastated. What had I done to deserve this, and why wasn't he prepared to help me?

I went to many other doctors for help. None would explain or diagnose my condition. Given the nature of my problem, it was humiliating having to go from doctor to doctor. Not only was the experience humiliating, but I couldn't help but feel that all were withholding information from me. Some made me feel like a child while others showed little empathy or concern. All I wanted was for someone to help me!

By the time I reached the sixth week of my recovery, my bladder was beginning to prolapse, causing a variety of other problems, and three months later, I experienced what is called a complete vaginal vault descent. In lay terms, this is a condition where the very top of the vagina descends to the exterior of a woman's body. The protrusion wasn't fixing itself, obviously, and I didn't want to have to live with this problem on a long-term basis. I don't know of any other woman who would have wanted to either.

Taking Charge

It became clear to me that I would have to help myself to medical information about my situation in order to have my problem addressed by specialists. I made many trips to the library of the medical school nearest my home, and I also began searching the Internet for other sources of information and support.

I had to do something. I no longer felt like a woman, sex was impossible and my hair started to fall out. The hot flashes and night sweats became unbearable, to the extent that I was feeling exhausted at all times. My breasts shrunk down to practically nothing, and I was beginning to think that this nightmare would never end.

I had no idea what to do next. The women I knew claimed that hysterectomy was as easy as getting a few stitches. They had no idea what I was going through. Finally, I found help from an online support group to which I belong to this day. It saddened me to learn through support groups that a great number of hysterectomized women suffer from sexual dysfunction. That's not what I read on the home care sheet that I was given when I left the hospital. It stated very clearly that hysterectomy would not affect my femininity or my sexuality.

Though most of the doctors I consulted insisted that my problems were all in my head, one didn't, and several months later, I underwent the first of many surgeries to correct the problems caused by my hysterectomy. I had to travel out of state for surgery on many occasions, and getting coverage for my health care proved difficult. This is a problem I will continue to encounter since prolapse repairs are not permanent fixes. These procedures will have to be repeated over time for the rest of my life.

It was hard to see what good could come out of all this, especially when a follow-up surgery caused nerve damage in my feet and I could no longer move my toes. The hysterectomy may have solved my problem with heavy periods, but the anemia and pelvic pain persisted. Years later, a specialist told me that my anemia was caused by a B12 vitamin shortage. And according to another specialist, my pelvic pain was apparently caused by muscular problems.

Neither my husband nor I can make any sense of all this, and no one could ever know the extent of our devastation. When we learned that my sexual dysfunction was permanent, my husband had a heart attack. This was such an overwhelming time for me that I wanted to die, too. Since my husband's recovery, we try to get through each day one at-a-time. Before my hysterectomy, my husband avoided being around sick people and hospitals, but since then, he became a pro at taking care of me and showing me that he still cares. I don't know what I'd do without him or my family.

Chere

❧

Hysterectomy seemed to be the only solution for me. I was not aware of other options. I was losing so much blood with my periods I became terrified that I would bleed to death. Since I was taking two birth control pills per day to control the hemorrhaging, I was willing to do anything to be normal again, including taking out the very parts that made me feel like a complete woman — my uterus and my cervix.

I sought a second opinion from a gynecologist and she agreed a hysterectomy would be an appropriate solution. She showed me a video of a woman who had a laparoscopic assisted vaginal hysterectomy (LAVH). The video showed the woman discussing the techniques of the surgery with her physician. Her physician, a male, was telling her all the positive outcomes of the surgery, including the importance of keeping her ovaries so she would continue to ovulate and produce her own hormones until she experienced menopause. Later, the video showed the woman discussing the outcome of her surgery. With enthusiasm, she described how well things had gone for her. She was excited, because she still had her ovaries and her sex life had *not* been negatively affected.

After viewing this video, I thought this surgery must be for me. No more periods, and no more worries about bleeding to death. Even though I had wanted to have another child, I would certainly never have to worry about birth control. Since I was keeping my ovaries, I would maintain my youthfulness, because I would still be ovulating and making my own hormones.

Confused by the Many Changes

My surgery went according to plan, but something about my body wasn't working right. I began to wonder what could have gone wrong. Only days after my surgery, I began having dizzy spells. It was difficult to stand without feeling vertigo. My body would sweat without cause, and my skin would become extremely flushed. My once oily complexion became very dry, and my curly hair began to thin and straighten. I would be overwhelmed with feelings of sadness and depression. I started having severe migraines so intense that I sought help from a neurologist.

My desire for sex disappeared; I had no desire to touch my husband and no desire to be touched by him. I was lethargic and constantly fatigued. My vision began to blur, and my memory began to challenge me. I was chairman of the board of a local non-profit agency, and I couldn't attend or conduct meetings without taking my husband along with me. I needed him to help me finish sentences or to jog my memory when it failed me. My once slender body weight of 119 during most of my adult life had jumped to 150 pounds, and I became ashamed of the way I looked. I no longer wanted to go out.

When I sought help from my gynecologist, she told me she couldn't find anything wrong with me. My blood test results indicated that my hormones were normal, and that my thyroid was within the acceptable range. She believed my problems were the result of a stressful work environment. She prescribed Zoloft, but it didn't help. I ended up leaving my job only to see my symptoms worsen.

Since my physician seemed satisfied with her conclusions, I needed more information about what was happening to me, and embarked on my own search for answers. I surfed the Web, and found other women experiencing some of the same symptoms. Like me, they were seeking support from other women. Their words sounded like an instant replay of a soundtrack of my own.

The Struggle with Weight

The weight gain had become a serious problem. Actually, I began gaining weight prior to my hysterectomy, because of the prescribed estrogen I was taking to control my heavy periods. When I went to the second gynecologist to seek advice about having a hysterectomy, she told me I would lose weight after the surgery. Shortly after the hysterectomy, I lost about three pounds, but gained these right back, and much more.

The unexplainable weight gain was a big issue for me, because throughout my life, people have always asked me if I was anorexic. In my early teens, a seamstress once told me I was the only person she knew who could stand behind a telephone pole, and no one would be able to see me. Even after having three full-term pregnancies, I remained skinny, and maintained a size four figure without dieting.

In 1996, when I began taking the pill to control the heavy bleeding, my weight went from approximately 119 to 142 pounds within a very short period of time. I couldn't purchase new clothing fast enough. In fact, there are still dresses in my closet that have never been worn, because I gained extra pounds before I could get into these. When I questioned my physicians about this, they simply laughed at me and replied: "Welcome to middle age." I had just turned 40.

I dieted. I starved. I worked out — even though sometimes I was so tired I could barely move from my couch to the chair in my living room. Nothing worked. I just kept gaining. Then one day I stepped on the scales only to be shocked by the sight of 160 pounds. These days, I fluctuate from 162 to 172, and I wear a size 14. I recently underwent more blood tests, and once again I was told that the hormones are normal and my thyroid is in the proper range (only now I know that the *proper* range was determined by thyroid tests conducted on males. I must admit that since I started on the Climara patch, I do feel a little better. But I still have the migraines, my sex life has become an occasional experience with short-lived orgasms that seem to stop as soon as they start, and my battle with weight gain is ongoing.

The Impact of Hysterectomy on my Career

My career has gone through many changes. Since the disabling migraines took control of my life, I am sometimes unable to leave my home. I stay home, because I can't think clearly, and my sight remains severely blurred. I sometimes feel extremely nauseous; I can't tolerate light and sound. During the last two years, I have sought treatment for snoring, a sleep disorder that many other women experience after having hysterectomies.

Last year, I spent the night in a clinic for sleep disorders. The results passed on to me by the doctor were laughable, because he didn't come up with anything I didn't know already. His written report showed that I was a 46-year-old female, I snored and I needed to lose weight.

I have found another more helpful pulmonologist. His view is that snoring and sleep apnea are problems associated with hormonal changes. Unfortunately, my medical insurance won't pay for his services. Research is now correlating strokes and heart disease with the loss of oxygen during sleep due to snoring and sleep apnea. So now I have one more thing to give me cause for concern.

With my symptoms, I could no longer work in the fast-paced and sometimes stressful corporate environment, so I had to find another career. In 2000, I returned to school and passed my state exams to become a Realtor. All those years I wasted at college working on a psychology degree and a Masters degree in communications! My new career enables me to work at my own pace; I work mainly from home, and I try to go about my daily activities regardless of the pain. I must survive, so I have learned to work around my limitations. My sex life is still next to nothing, and my husband has learned to accept it. I used to enjoy seeing an attractive man. Now I don't even bother to look.

I realize that many of the symptoms I'm experiencing occur gradually during menopause. But my menopause occurred immediately after the removal of my uterus and my cervix. I wasn't prepared for the sudden change.

If I had to do it all over again, I would not. I would seek other opinions. I would find other physicians who would give me options, and who be willing to work with me to find the best possible alternative treatment for me and for my body. Of course, I can't change what has been done, but I can share my experiences with others considering this life-altering surgery. I can talk to others about my lost dreams and my adjusted lifestyle. For the record, my experience is not one I would want for my daughter. This is one future I don't want to have in common with my beautiful girl.

Mary Anne

❧

Mary Anne Wyatt is the author of the overview that introduces this section. From the beginning, I told her that this work would not be complete without her help. Her research into the history of hysterec-tomy and its consequences has proved invaluable to Misinformed Consent. *It was an honour and a pleasure for me to work with someone so dedicated to making a difference for hysterectomized women all over the world.*

In 1993, a year before my surgery, the low, dull, cramping pain that sometimes lasted through my monthly cycle was diagnosed as a symptomatic fibroid, or benign uterine tumour. I was approaching menopause, and skipping every third period on average. I didn't suffer from premenstrual syndrome, and I hadn't had pain for six months before my surgery. My posture was straight, and I had only a soft roll of fat just above the pubic hairline. I took pride in my pear-shaped body, with its larger hips, smaller waist, and flat abdomen from years of intense physical activity. I had skated competitively into my forties, was an avid mountain climber, and went on adventurous flying trips into environmentally protected areas. I walked five miles a day until the day before the surgery.

I felt terrific. My life was full of plans — for orchestra playing, travel abroad, and graduate work. I was a single woman with an active social life who performed frequently as a jazz musician. I loved being female, wearing pretty clothes, flirting, and having intimate relationships with men. I never once questioned the possibility of losing it all.

"I Am Scheduling Your Hysterectomy"

Shortly after my gynecologist discovered the fibroid tumour in a routine exam, she called me to say, "I am scheduling your hysterectomy." At the follow-up appointment she said she thought I had cancer. When I challenged both her decision and diagnosis, and told her that I didn't want a hysterectomy without proof of existing pathology, she slammed the door on me, leaving me alone in her office to ponder her words in shock. Gathering my strength, I opened the door and followed her into the hallway.

"Why do you think I have cancer?" I asked.

"Because you're still menstruating," she answered.

Her reasoning was both absurd and frightening, and unsupported by the endometrial biopsy I had subsequently. Done to determine whether I had endometrial cancer, it was clearly negative.

I began a quest, booking a series of appointments with other gynecologists and at the same time researching alternatives to hysterectomy. Myomectomy was one alternative that was gaining media attention at the time. There was still no certainty that I needed surgery at all. I could have waited until menopause, when the fibroid would shrink of its own accord. I decided, however, that I wanted a myomectomy.

I found two doctors in the Boston area who had the qualifications to perform a myomectomy. Gynecologists and other experts emphasized the importance of having a highly experienced and expert surgeon to perform either myomectomy or hysterectomy, to avoid potential injury to the uterus, muscles, urinary tract, and other pelvic structures. I chose a gynecologist who had published on fibroids, had the necessary skill, and who operated at a large teaching hospital, which seemed to me the safest place to be in the event of complications. He was also board-certified in endocrinology. I trusted him.

The gynecologist examined me only once, very briefly. He said that the likelihood of my developing uterine cancer was slim. After measuring my FSH (follicle-stimulating hormone) level to determine that I was premenopausal, he offered to include me in a study he was conducting on Lupron. I declined, however, when he told me that the fibroid would return if I stopped taking the drug, and because of its possible side effects. Because I had a fibroid, he told me, hormone replacement therapy (HRT) would not be an option for me after surgery: Fibroids grow faster when they are exposed to estrogen, including the estrogen found in HRT.

The gynecologist did not recommend a myomectomy. In fact, he argued against it, telling me that my uterus would never return to a normal size after he removed the fibroid. (Later, another specialist told me that this was simply a lie. I have come to believe that the gynecologist was trying to push me into having a hysterectomy.) I had no reason not to trust him, and I reluctantly agreed to the hysterectomy.

If a hysterectomy was necessary, I requested that the doctor remove only my uterus, leaving my ovaries intact with a good blood supply, and leaving my cervix for the purpose of lubrication and structural support of the bladder. To help explain my requests, I brought Dr. Winnifred B. Cutler's book *Hysterectomy Before and After* to my doctor's appointments and discussed the specific citations in the book regarding ovarian and cervical function. (The gynecologist did agree to leave my other organs intact, but he left only a small remnant of my cervix and my ovaries, which ceased functioning almost immediately.)

I cared deeply about both the appearance of my body and my sex life, and I emphasized those concerns repeatedly to the gynecologist.

I did not want an ugly vertical incision, and I was concerned about what I had read about hysterectomy destroying a woman's sex life. Finally the doctor told me that he would make a Pfannenstiel (bikini-line) incision to maintain the appearance of my body. But apparently he thought that sexual arousal and bodily pleasure were all in the head. "Don't worry," he said. "I'm not operating on your brain."

The Deception Begins

During my appointments with the gynecologist, I insisted that no resident was to perform my hysterectomy. In response, he stood up, put his fists on the table, and exclaimed emphatically, "No one touches my patients but me!" His answer gave me complete confidence that he would perform all of the surgery.

I also told him that I wanted an epidural anesthetic, which would allow me to stay awake during the operation. He agreed to the epidural, but told me to discuss it with a friend he recommended in the hospital's anesthesiology department.

Finally, I asked for a video of the surgery, so that I would know that no residents had operated on me. My request was refused. "We don't do that here," said my doctor. I also requested a pre-surgery hormonal blood profile so that I could compare it to my hormone levels after hysterectomy. If I did experience side effects, I reasoned, it would then be easier to supplement my body with the right mixture of hormones. Once more, I was declined.

At my last doctor's appointment before the hysterectomy, I was rushed into signing a blank consent form on the way out of the office, and then rushed into pre-operative testing before closing time.

I repeatedly attempted to make an appointment with the anesthesiologist at the hospital. During my telephone conversations with her, I told her how important it was that no resident operated on me. Since she lived nearby, she suggested coming over to my house, in lieu of meeting at the hospital, to talk to me about the anesthesia. However, she repeatedly put me off. Finally, two nights before the surgery, she called to say that the gynecologist had changed his mind and wanted to use general anesthesia. When I objected, she said that I could discuss the issue with him or change doctors. "He has his reasons," she said.

I attempted numerous times to reach her and discuss the anesthesia, but she returned none of my calls. On the day of the operation, I tried to call the surgeon, but he didn't answer my calls either. Lying on the operating table, I was still expecting to speak to the surgeon before the operation. The anesthesiologist said to me in passing, "Don't be concerned if you see me next to someone else." I was terrified. I could see the gynecologist on the other side, but no one else. I tried again to talk to him, but he interrupted me by signalling to the anesthesiologist. I immediately lost consciousness. After the surgery, I never saw the anesthesiologist again.

After Surgery

I awoke to find myself arched on the hospital bed, unable to lie down flat. No position was comfortable. My abdomen protruded straight out from my body at least five inches more than it had before surgery. The medical personnel attributed this development to post-surgical swelling. The roll of fat was gone, and the incision area was flat. Intense, sharp, fleeting pains shot through my pelvis. I couldn't sleep.

On the second day after surgery, a resident came to see me. He told me that he, not my gynecologist, had performed the surgery. When I asked why I hadn't been given an epidural, he said that he didn't like them because a patient on an epidural had once kicked him. Panic, fear, and anger seized me as I realized that I had been betrayed — and also that something was terribly wrong with my body. The resident couldn't answer many of my questions, yet he admitted to having done the surgery. I couldn't believe that this situation hadn't been premeditated by the entire operating team.

Further alarms went off in my head when the resident told me he didn't know how to use the staple-remover to remove the surgical staples. It was a Friday and he was alone, so he asked me to help. Unfortunately, I was unable to see over my belly to do as he requested. I wondered what would happen if the stitches didn't hold, but together we were finally able to finish the job successfully.

I asked for both my records and the pathology report, only to be told that they were unavailable. When I was discharged, the only orders I had were to go home and walk.

More Problems, Fewer Answers

After two weeks, I was still unable to lie flat or sleep for longer than five hours. The centre of my body still protruded so much that I looked pregnant. Inside, I felt an awful, uncomfortable pressure. I began to notice tremors in my left hand. Six weeks after the surgery, I experienced a deep and lasting pain with orgasm.

For more than two months I couldn't get my records or an appointment to see the gynecologist. During that time, his substitute examined me, but he ignored my questions about pain and the abdominal protrusion. "It will go down," he said. He did not address my orgasmic pain, lack of sleep, loss of libido, or difficulty standing up straight and lying down flat.

Six weeks after the surgery, I received a call from a nurse at the hospital. When I told her of my increasing pain and symptoms, she dismissed them. "Dr. X's patients don't have problems!" she said. (Later I was told that serious complications can arise from refusal to diagnose and treat hysterectomy-related pain at the outset.)

When I finally saw my surgeon, I asked him outright, "Who did the surgery?"

"I did," he answered. I did not challenge him, but I knew otherwise.

He refused to examine me. He wrote "abdominal protrusion" in my file, and left me with the pat, unsatisfactory explanation that he had "pulled everything up." Still I had no answers.

For my difficulty sleeping, the gynecologist referred me to a specialist at the hospital's sleep clinic, where I was diverted to a psychologist. He interrogated me twice, but refused to acknowledge that my problems might be related to the hysterectomy. Instead, he asked irrelevant questions about my early childhood. I did not go back to the sleep clinic; it was obvious to me that they felt the problem was "all in my head."

Desperate for knowledge about what had happened to me, tired, and in pain, I attended meditation classes with Jon Kabat-Zinn, a compassionate and deeply caring individual. His teaching helped me to continue living within a body that, by then, I wished had gone to the morgue the day of my operation.

Struggling for Answers

Gradually, my pain with orgasm increased to the point where I found it impossible to have sex. The pain had become diffuse and predominant on my left side, from beneath my urethra into my left groin, buttock, and low back. Walking, standing, or lying down for more than fifteen minutes in one position became impossible. Seeking relief from the low back pain, I bent over when I walked, like a much older woman. I couldn't lie on my back. In fact, no sleeping position was comfortable. The constant pain and lack of sleep were turning me into an invalid.

In addition to the chronic pain, abdominal protrusion, severe loss of sleep, and tremors in my hand, I also had endocrine (hormonal) problems. My formerly thick, curly hair was now straight and thinning. I was gaining weight, and I had lost sexual desire. As well, I was beginning to fall when I walked, tumbling forward because my left leg and hip wouldn't work in concert with the right side of my body. Eventually I fell while carrying a glass bottle, severing an artery and nerves in my left hand — my music career as a string player was over.

In order to survive, I had to address all these problems. I sought out the opinions of many doctors in various specialties. Within several months of the surgery, I saw a noted urologist, who identified a pelvic nerve injury from the hysterectomy. Eight months after the surgery, an expert in surgical plastic reconstruction finally diagnosed a "mistake," and said she could repair my abdomen. Another told me I had a separation in my abdominal muscles "four or five inches wide," and a third said that my abdomen was herniated and prolapsed, or sagging, because of a lack of muscle and ligament support.

Finally, Help

My initial fleeting pains had increased steadily until they became chronic, and eventually intolerable. I was sent by a urologist to a pain clinic for a possible lidocaine infusion and narcotics, but soon rejected the therapy when I realized that I would once again be at the mercy of residents who weren't well versed in how to treat pelvic nerve injury. I left, grateful to have received a small quantity of pain-relieving drugs.

On the verge of hopelessness, I found an excellent pelvic-floor specialist who worked with a urogynecologist in Chicago. Through my vaginal wall, they could easily palpate the damaged structures, rigid muscles, and other soft tissues that were contributing to my pelvic-floor muscle pain. Their evaluation showed severe lordosis (abnormal curvature) of the spine, multiple trigger points (tight knots of tissue) in my pelvic-floor muscles, and severe muscle and soft tissue pain.

Upon examining me, the therapist exclaimed, "Oh my God, they got your psoas!"

The psoas is a large muscle that connects the lower spine to the thighbone and gives stability to the spine. Prolonged compression from incorrect use of surgical retractors in a hysterectomy can injure both the psoas and the pelvic nerves that run through it. Severe lordosis can result from a combination of poor positioning during surgery and extreme trauma to the muscles and nerves. To address these problems, my therapy would be extensive, requiring trigger-point injections of the drug Marcaine into the pelvic-floor muscles, to be given by a surgeon with a working knowledge of pelvic-floor anatomy.

The pelvic-floor specialist also said that general anesthesia had been a bad choice, since it leaves muscles unprotected and more subject to trauma. I was told that no one should have been left with my symptoms. Moreover, prompt, intensive physical therapy soon after the surgery might have saved me from a lifetime of constant pain.

I spent more than $45,000 for out-of-pocket medical expenses in 1996 alone, mostly for pain relief therapy. With continual muscular and trigger-point therapy and stretching exercises, I have been able to partially relieve my pain. The lordosis has improved from severe to moderate, but my pelvis is still twisted by muscle contraction, and my back pain remains. I was prescribed a heavy plastic back brace. As I write this, I face possible spinal fusion surgery. The protrusion in my abdomen has not "gone down," as the gynecologist's substitute told me it would. I still have insomnia. And I avoid sexual activity because it is too painful.

Validation — and Survival

In 1996, a friend sent me a Federal Register report about findings of scientific misconduct. The report stated that the gynecologist who had performed my surgery had falsified data in published research (including the study he had asked me to join) and had also falsified patients' records for those studies. Eventually his medical license was suspended.

When I read the report, I felt validated. The enormous burden of proof had been lifted from me. This discovery, although upsetting in its own right, was a necessary part of my healing. I no longer had to scream into the wind that I had been wronged. Perhaps others would now come forward and a physician would help me with my pain. My friends and family could support me openly.

At present, I try to live from one moment to the next, in a vastly different and more spiritual persona than my pre-hysterectomy self. My physical body is frequently in great pain, and my mind must cope with the results of this terrible deceit and betrayal. I am grateful for the many friends I have met who are suffering from similar circumstances, who encourage my fighting, activist spirit, and who believe in me. I am equally grateful to those who introduced me to the practice of meditation. I thank the doctors and therapists who dared to tell me the truth, and who have helped me get proper medical diagnoses and led me to treatment options. Gradually, I am learning to trust myself.

PART III

Resources

Publications of Interest

Hysterectomy and Oophorectomy

Hysterectomy Before and After: A Comprehensive Guide to Preventing, Preparing for, and Maximizing Health After Hysterectomy
Winnifred B. Cutler, Ph.D. (Harper Perennial, 1988) ISBN 0060159162

Many American women are not aware of the long-term consequences of hysterectomy and the full range of alternative treatments available. This book is based on a review of more than 3,500 recent studies as well as research conducted by the author, reproductive biologist Dr. Winnifred Cutler. Dr. Cutler uses clear language to explain all aspects of hysterectomy, including new evidence showing the vital role of the uterus and ovaries to a woman's well-being. She explains why hysterectomy should be avoided in most cases, when it must be performed, and how the patient's health can be restored and maintained after surgery.

Dr. Winnifred Cutler is the President of the Athena Institute for Women's Wellness, Inc., in Chester Springs, Pennsylvania. She is a graduate of the University of Pennsylvania who went on to do postdoctoral work at Stanford University, where she established the Stanford Menopause Study. Dr. Cutler is the co-founder of the Women's Wellness Program at the Hospital of the University of Pennsylvania. She has co-authored five other books and her research has been featured in many U.S. publications.

Hysterectomy and Ovary Removal: What ALL Women Need to KNOW
Elizabeth L. Plourde, CLS, MA (New Voice Publications, 2001) ISBN
0966173538

This book is the culmination of sixteen years of research into more than
forty-five thousand medical journal articles. In an easily understandable
format, it presents vital information for women about the functions of
the uterus, ovaries, and hormones. Elizabeth wrote *Hysterectomy and
Ovary Removal* expressly for

- women facing the decision of whether to undergo hysterectomy for
  non–life-threatening conditions and/or prophylactic ovarian removal;
- hysterectomized women with no symptoms or who are suffering from
  surgical consequences;
- women who have undergone ovarian removal;
- women making decisions about hormone replacement.

*Elizabeth Plourde is a licensed clinical laboratory scientist with a BS
in Biological Science and an MA in psychology. Her training in the fields
of medicine and psychology has been augmented by a decade's worth of
work with cutting-edge cancer and genetics medical research laboratories.
With* Hysterectomy and Ovary Removal, *Elizabeth Plourde has written
the book she wishes had been available before she said yes to this
irreversible, life-changing operation.*

The Case Against Hysterectomy
Sandra Simkin (Pandora, 1996) ISBN 0044409788

*Sandra Simkin worked in public relations for blue-chip companies for
twelve years and planned to set up a PR consultancy in 1993, the same
year she was pressured into having a hysterectomy/oophorectomy. She
agreed to the surgery only because the possibility of ovarian cancer
was grossly overstated. One year later, she found out that the operation
had been unnecessary. In 1995 she founded the Campaign Against*

Hysterectomy and Unnecessary Operations on Women, a pressure group aimed at achieving a Women's Medical Protection Act to set limitations on doctors. Elected to Woking Borough Council in May 1996, she served as councillor until April 2000. In 1996 she was also elected to the North West Surrey Community Health Council.

The Castrated Woman: What Your Doctor Won't Tell You About Hysterectomy
Naomi Miller Stokes (Franklin Watts, 1986) ISBN 0531150038

Naomi Miller Stokes gives readers an excellent overview of the many side effects that can result from hysterectomy. Her focus is on sexual dysfunction and loss of libido, and the tremendous impact it can have on relationships. Disturbed by the wall of silence she faced when she asked questions about her own post-hysterectomy difficulties, she embarked on a massive investigation, interviewing over 500 doctors, psychiatrists, and women patients to get the answers she was looking for. The end result was this moving book about truth and survival as a castrated woman.

The Hysterectomy Hoax
Stanley T. West, M.D., with Paula Dranov (originally published by Doubleday in 1994). New edition to be released in April 2002 by Next Decade, Inc. ISBN 0970090811

More than 600,000 hysterectomies are performed each year in the United States. Only 10% of them are necessary, argues Dr. Stanley West, a leading New York physician and surgeon and the chief of the Division of Reproductive Endocrinology & Infertility at St. Vincent's Hospital and Medical Center. Dr. West explains why hysterectomies are often the surgeon's recommended choice and provides the information necessary for women to make informed decisions regarding their options.

In *The Hysterectomy Hoax*, Dr. West takes a firm stand against the surgery except in cases where a woman has cancer. In fact, he persuasively argues that the surgery can do more harm than good and presents unnecessary risks, except in those situations involving a life-threatening illness. In almost every other case, there is an alternative treatment or surgery that avoids hysterectomy.

Dr. West minces no words in his criticism of his colleagues for taking the "easy way out" by performing hysterectomies as a panacea for a wide range of conditions, from PMS to uterine fibroids and endometriosis. He further explains how insurance companies contribute to the high rate of hysterectomy in the United States. But more importantly, the author empowers women to take control of their health care by explaining how their bodies work and providing the questions they should ask their doctors before agreeing to this surgery. He believes that a "well-informed" woman, who has an understanding of her body, is at an enormous advantage.

Christina Ferrare Discusses Sexual Desire
Transcript of *The Oprah Winfrey Show*, January 15, 1998 (Harpo Productions, Inc.). Transcript produced by Burrelle's Information Services, P.O. Box 7, Livingston, NJ 07039. To obtain a copy, call 1-800-7777-TEXT (8398).

Christina Ferrare and Judith Reichman, M.D., discuss loss of sexual desire and drive after total abdominal hysterectomy and bilateral salpingo-oophorectomy.

What Women Are Saying About Hysterectomy
Transcript of *The Oprah Winfrey Show*, July 15, 1998 (Harpo Productions, Inc.). Transcript produced by Burrelle's Information Services, P.O. Box 7, Livingston, NJ 07039. To obtain a copy, call 1-800-7777-TEXT (8398).

Judith Reichman, M.D., of Los Angeles, author of *I'm Too Young to Get Old*, discusses the many side effects of hysterectomy.

Menopause

The Menopause, HRT and You
Caroline Hawkridge (Penguin, 1999) ISBN 0140272615

This book is for women of all ages. It includes up-to-date information on natural and surgical menopause, hormonal replacement therapy, osteoporosis, breast cancer, and heart disease.

A Woman Doctor's Guide to Menopause
Lois Jovanovic, M.D., with Suzanne LeVert (Hyperion, 1993)
ISBN 156282855X

Dr. Lois Jovanovic is a leading endocrinologist, and her book is a comprehensive guide for women looking for information on natural menopause and premature menopause caused by hysterectomy. She tackles all the issues from hot flashes to changes in sex drive as well as the pros and cons of hormone replacement therapy.

The Silent Passage: Menopause
Gail Sheehy (Pocket Books, 1998) ISBN 0671799312

Gail Sheehy's landmark bestseller has become the bible for women concerned about menopause (including surgical menopause). In the years since *The Silent Passage* was originally published, the author, a member of the Health Advisory Committee to the Women's Health Initiative, has been at the forefront of research on menopause. She has also continued to interview countless women on the subject. In this revised and expanded edition, she presents essential new data that will enable women to custom-design their own hormone replacement regimes.

What Your Doctor May Not Tell You About Menopause:
The Breakthrough Book on Natural Progesterone
John R. Lee, M.D., with Virginia Hopkins (Warner Books, 1996)
ISBN 0446671444

John R. Lee, M.D., has pioneered work in women's health and is the
author of *Natural Progesterone*. Recently retired from private practice
after thirty years, he now teaches medical professionals and lay
audiences about hormone balance and health.

Dr. Lee's book provides exciting facts about natural progesterone and
how it can deliver what HRT and estrogen only promise. Premenopausal
symptoms, endometriosis, weight gain, low sex drive, fibrocystic breasts,
heart disease, and osteoporosis — most women will experience these or
other hormone-related problems. Today, millions of women concerned
about aging must decide whether to undergo synthetic hormone replacement therapy — and suffer its side effects and increased risk of cancer —
or not.

However, there is revolutionary news about completely safe, natural
progesterone, the only hormone supplement women may need as they
age. In his book Dr. Lee brings you lifesaving facts that even your doctor
may not know about Premarin, Provera, and other HRT drugs; outlines
an easy-to-follow non-prescription "hormone balance" program; and
tells you how to stay energized, strong, sexually vigorous, and free from
"female problems" before menopause, during the menopausal years,
and beyond. This book also includes sections on why hysterectomy
should be avoided unless cancer has been detected.

Is It HOT in Here or Is It Me?
Gayle Sand, with a foreword by Morris Notelovits, M.D., Ph.D.
(Harper Spotlight, 1993) ISBN 0061093572

This is an interesting book on natural menopause. Gayle Sand discusses
intimate, enlightening and amusing details about her personal experience, and provides good facts on alternative hormonal treatments.

Hormone Function and Hormone Replacement Therapy

The HRT Solution: Restoring Your Vitality, Sexuality and Health Through an Individualized Hormone Replacement Program
Marla Ahlgrimm, RPH, and John M. Kells (Avery, a division of Penguin Putnam, Inc., 1999) ISBN 0895299488

This is an excellent book! From it, women will learn in simplified language all there is to know about their hormones and hormone replacement therapy. Women considering HRT may find that the information they receive is often confusing and inconclusive. One day we're told that estrogen protects women from Alzheimer's disease, the next, that it causes breast cancer. Some women say HRT makes them feel terrific; others who try it experience side effects, or no effects at all. Many women instinctively resist taking synthetic or animal-derived hormones because they seem unnatural.

In *The HRT Solution*, Marla Ahlgrimm and John Kells explain what hormones are, how they work, and how they affect virtually every aspect of life. Most importantly, the authors introduce a revolutionary approach to hormone management that combines simple but precise testing to monitor hormone levels, and individualized doses of natural hormones that are identical to those made by the body. In addition to "recharging batteries" and relieving menopausal symptoms, natural hormone replacement can help stop bone loss and protect the heart and brain from the degenerative processes commonly associated with aging. With an individualized approach to hormone replacement, women can finally understand their hormones and bring them back to their proper balance.

The Truth about Hormone Replacement Therapy: How to Break Free from the Medical Myths of Menopause
National Women's Health Network (Prima Publishing, 2002) ISBN 0-7615-3478-4

This book discloses the major health risks associated with hormone replacement therapy (HRT), with the objective of helping women make informed decisions about HRT, for the relief of symptoms associated with natural or surgical menopause. It also offers information on natural alternatives.

The Women's Health Network, a collective of doctors and researchers, analyzed studies done on HRT for menopause, and concluded that HRT is a "triumph of marketing over science and advertising over common sense".

According to the authors, effective marketing has convinced women and many health care practitioners that menopause is a disease that must be treated with pharmaceuticals, and that HRT can prevent such major illnesses as heart disease, colon cancer and Alzheimer's. Hormones are often prescribed as preventatives, despite the lack of evidence to support their effectiveness in this role. However, HRT does carry the risk of serious side effects, including certain cancers.

The Truth about Hormone Replacement Therapy will help women to decide if they should take such risky drugs to help them deal with menopause.

Screaming to Be Heard: Hormonal Connections Women Suspect and Doctors Ignore
Elizabeth Lee Vliet, M.D. (M. Evans and Company, 1995) ISBN 0871317842

This volume of 500-plus pages contains a mountain of information, described by the author as "the tapestry woven of women's experiences as I listened to them over my twenty years in medicine." This encyclopedia of "overlooked and ignored hormonal connections that interact at all levels in women's health" provides solid information about the connection between the body and the mind.

In addition to two decades' of experience as a physician, Dr. Vliet brings her personal commitment to the information in *Screaming to Be Heard*: "I have not made any recommendations or any interpretations from the medical literature that I would not use myself for my own health needs or recommend to my own family to consider with their physicians." With that kind of backing, readers can turn to *Screaming to Be Heard* with confidence as they seek information about options for dealing with everything from chronic fatigue to weight problems to migraines.

Dr. Vliet is the founder of HER Place, the Women's Center for Health Enhancement and Renewal in Tucson, Arizona, and Fort Worth, Texas (www.herplace.com).

Premenstrual Syndrome (PMS)

Once a Month: The Original Premenstrual Syndrome Handbook
4th edition, Katharina Dalton, M.D. (Hunter House, 1999) ISBN 0897930711. To order, please call 1-800-266-5592, fax 510-865-4295, visit our Web site at **www.hunterhouse.com**, or write to Hunter House Publishers, PO Box 2914, Alameda, CA 94501.

First published in 1979, *Once a Month* was the breakthrough book that introduced an American audience to the definition of premenstrual syndrome and how it can be controlled. Women can often treat common PMS symptoms themselves. In severe cases, progesterone therapy under medical supervision can be immediately effective.

The fourth edition of *Once a Month*

- explains clearly the two different types of menstrual cramps, and which type is a PMS symptom;
- includes a chapter addressed to men whose wives, daughters, partners, or friends are severely affected by PMS;
- offers clear explanations of post-hysterectomy and post-oophorectomy depression as it relates to PMS; (Although it is true that PMS symptoms often require drastic treatment, hysterectomy is *not* the answer. According to Dalton's research, PMS always increases in severity after a hysterectomy, whether or not the ovaries have been removed.)
- includes a full report on findings about progesterone receptor sites in the body. (The discovery that these receptors are inhibited by certain

chemicals, including possibly adrenaline, may lead us to the *real* cause of premenstrual syndrome.)

Dr. Dalton is the foremost authority on PMS and its treatment. In 1953 she co-authored the first medical paper on premenstrual syndrome. Shortly thereafter, she established the world's first PMS clinic in London, England, where for over thirty years she treated more than forty thousand women. Her books and papers are currently published worldwide in twelve languages.

Health Care for Women

Our Bodies, Ourselves for the New Century: A Book by and for Women
Boston Women's Health Book Collective (Simon & Schuster, 1998)
ISBN 0684842319.
To order a copy online, go to **www.bwhbc.org/obos.htm**.

Our Bodies, Ourselves for the New Century reflects the vital health concerns of women of diverse ages, ethnic and racial backgrounds, and sexual orientations. In these pages, women will find new information, resources (including Internet resources), and personal support for the decisions that will shape their health — and their lives. The topics explored range from living a healthy life, relationships, sexuality, childbearing, and growing older, to dealing with the medical system and organizing for change. This is a book for women of all generations to use, rely on, and share with others.

I'm Too Young to Get Old: Health Care for Women After Forty
Judith Reichman, M.D. (Random House, 1996) ISBN 0812924258;
I'm NOT in the Mood: What Every Woman Should Know About Improving Her Libido
Judith Reichman, M.D. (Quill, 1999) ISBN 0688172253

In *I'm Too Young to Get Old*, Dr. Judith Reichman speaks frankly about the most pressing health concerns of today's older women. She discusses contraception, fertility, and pregnancy after forty; menopause; and hormone replacement therapy and nonmedical alternatives.

I'm NOT in the Mood deals with the issue of loss of sexual desire following hysterectomy. Judith Reichman outlines when it's time to see a psychiatrist, psychologist, or sex therapist and the seven things that can sabotage your libido. *I'm NOT in the Mood* outlines how to talk to your doctor about sexual disorders, how to reach your biological sexual potential, and what can be of help.

Judith Reichman, M.D., practises and teaches at Cedars-Sinai Medical Center and UCLA in Los Angeles. She wrote and co-hosted the acclaimed PBS series Straight Talk on Menopause *and* More Straight Talk on Menopause. *She appears regularly on the* Today Show *as a contributor on women's health issues.*

Other Publications of Interest

Fibromyalgia, A Comprehensive Approach: What You Can Do About Chronic Pain and Fatigue
Miryam Ehrlich Williamson (Walker and Co., 1996) ISBN 0802774849;
The Fibromyalgia Relief Book: 213 Ideas for Improving Your Quality of Life
Miryam Ehrlich Williamson (Walker and Co., 1996) ISBN 0802775535

Distressing as it is, fibromyalgia is not life-threatening and it need not worsen over time. If you, or someone you know, suffers from the symptoms of fibromyalgia syndrome (FMS), such as muscular stiffness, disturbed sleep, and fatigue, help yourself to the information in *Fibromyalgia: A Comprehensive Approach*.

For those with fibromyalgia, *The Fibromyalgia Relief Book* is about making life more liveable at home, at work, while travelling or socializing, and in your personal relationships. There's a section devoted to diet and nutrition, because the author firmly believes that the way we eat has a great deal to do with how we feel. There is also a section on resources and a step-by-step method for taking control of your health. For additional information on how to get your fibromyalgia under control, visit Miryam's Web site at **www.mwilliamson.com**.

Miryam Williamson is a medical and technical journalist who has had fibromyalgia since early childhood.

Eating Well, Living Well with Osteoporosis
Connie W. Bales, Ph.D., RD, Marc K. Drezner, M.D., and Kimberly P. Hoben, RD, MPH, LDN (Penguin Books, 1996) ISBN 0670866598

This book is about dietary approaches to healthy living for women who have undergone hysterectomies and/or oophorectomies, and who have doubled their risk of osteoporosis because of the surgical removal of their ovaries.

Endometriosis: A Key to Healing Through Nutrition
Dian Shepperson Mills and Michael Walter Vernon (Element Books, 1999) ISBN 1862043000

The following is an excerpt from this book:

> Endometriosis is not as easy as measles or a broken leg to treat. It is a systemic disease, and it may be an auto-immune disorder. We have to correct the cause of the disease, but we are unsure how it originates, so our only defense against it must be by attempting to regain our health through a healthy diet, rest and gentle exercise. Women need to listen to the messages their body gives them. Illness is an imbalance and good nutrition can help redress that imbalance.

For more information about this book, visit **www.obgyn.net/endo/ articles/nutrient.htm**.

Progesterone in Orthomolecular Medicine
Ray Peat, Ph.D.
This book discusses the use of progesterone as it relates to hormone imbalances, and also describes some common signs and symptoms of thyroid and progesterone deficiencies.

Generative Energy: Protecting and Restoring the Wholeness of Life
Ray Peat, Ph.D.
This book provides the general scientific and biological information that makes possible a nutritional and therapeutic reorientation.

Mind and Tissue: Russian Research Perspectives on the Human Brain
Ray Peat, Ph.D.
This book offers new perspectives for expanding our scientific traditions.

Nutrition for Women
Ray Peat, Ph.D.
This book contains ninety-two short articles focusing on topics pertaining to women's health, for example, pregnancy, weight gain, weight loss, arthritis, nutrition and hormones, premenstrual tension, menopause, and stress.

From PMS to Menopause: Female Hormones in Context
Ray Peat, Ph.D.
Scientifically understanding the subject of female sexuality and health means going against the currents of both conventional and alternative medicine. This book considers in detail a variety of problem areas affecting women from childhood to old age.

Dr. Peat has a Ph.D. in biology from the University of Oregon, with specialization in physiology. He has taught at the University of Oregon, Urbana College, Montana State University, the National College of Naturopathic Medicine, Universidad Veracruzana, Universidad Autonoma del Estado de Mexico, and Blake College. Currently he also conducts private counselling sessions on nutrition.

Dr. Peat started his work with progesterone and related hormones in 1968. In his papers on physiological chemistry and physics (1971 and 1972) and in his dissertation (University of Oregon, 1972), he outlined his ideas regarding progesterone and the hormones closely related to it as protectors of the body's structure and energy against the harmful effects of estrogen, radiation, stress, and lack of oxygen.

*To order these books, contact Dr. Peat at P.O. Box 5764, Eugene, OR 97405, or on the Internet at **www.efn.org/~raypeat/**.*

Medical Schools, Health Care Systems, and the Pharmaceutical Industry

Kill or Cure? How Canadians Can Remake Their Health Care System

Carolyn Bennett, M.D., and Rick Archbold (HarperCollins, 2000) ISBN 000639101X

Dr. Carolyn Bennett is well qualified to assess Canada's health care system. A family physician and founding partner of Bedford Medical Associates, she is the federal member of Parliament for St. Paul's riding in Toronto. Until her election, she was president of the Medical Staff Association of Women's College Hospital. She is an assistant professor in the Department of Family and Community Medicine at the University of Toronto. Dr. Bennett was the host of Doctor on Call *on the Women's Television Network, and is a frequent media commentator on health care issues in Canada. She lives with her family in Toronto.*

The Drug Lords: America's Pharmaceutical Cartel

Tonda R. Bian (No Barriers Publishing, 1997) ISBN 0965456803
To order, call 1-800-828-3057 or visit
www.askthenutritiondoctor.com.

Tens of thousands of people die each year from drugs their doctors prescribe for them. Tens of thousands more experience debilitating side effects. Yet Americans are consuming drugs faster than ever — all with the misguided belief that drugs heal. The truth is, most drugs do not heal, but only mask the symptoms of illness and disease. More seriously, many commonly used drugs have been found to cause health- and life-threatening conditions that range from depression to death. Still, most people are convinced that there is a pill for whatever ails them. This is the lie that has turned us into a society of pharmaceutical junkies. *The Drug Lords* shoots a critical look at our overprescribed, overmedicated society and the role that the pharmaceutical industry plays in keeping us that way.

Tonda Bian has worked as a consumer advocate, investigative reporter, and corporate communications specialist. She became interested in the dangers of over-the-counter and prescription drugs after realizing that her own health problems were likely the result of a prescription drug her mother took during pregnancy. After seeing first-hand the failures of traditional medical treatments, Tonda is now an advocate for alternative and complementary healing. She is currently involved in developing a syndicated newspaper column entitled "Health Tracks," which is designed to follow political developments in health care.

Heart Failure: Diary of a Third-Year Medical Student
Michael Greger, M.D., and United Progressive Alumni (Cornell University, 1999) ISBN 0967828813

In 1999, Michael Greger, M.D., graduated with honours from the Tufts University School of Medicine. While in his third year (a critical year in medical education), Dr. Greger kept a detailed diary of everything that he saw and experienced. He had viewed medicine as a humanistic career of helping people, sharing, and caring for people. However, what he found was a profession that did not even seem to care *about* people. Why did he write it all down? For Dr. Greger, it was a way to get medical school out of his system, but also a way to make sure he would never forget.

All profits from the sale of this book go to charity. To order, call (617) 524-8064, send an e-mail to **mhg1@cornell.edu**, or visit the Web site at **www.upalumni.org/medschool**.

The Unkindest Cut: Life in the Backrooms of Medicine

Marcia Millman (Morrow Quill Paperbacks, 1977) ISBN 0688081207

This book offers a description and analysis of some of the "backrooms" of American medicine — a look at what is said and done in operating rooms, at mortality review conferences, in the emergency room, and at various kinds of hospital staff meetings. The focus of the book is on features of the everyday world of the hospital that adversely affect the quality of patient care. This book goes right to the heart of hospital life: the behaviour, conflicts, and competition among doctors, and how errors and incompetence are covered up. It is based on sociologist Marcia Millman's two-year study of daily life in several hospitals.

Operating in the Dark: The Accountability Crisis in Canada's Health Care System

Lisa Priest (Doubleday Canada, 1998) ISBN 0385257198

In *Operating in the Dark*, journalist Lisa Priest goes behind the green curtain and into the nation's hospitals to ask tough questions about how accountable our cherished medical system really is. With investigative skill, she puts a human face to the charts and the caseloads. From questionable surgery rates for hysterectomy to overprescribed drugs, women have specific concerns regarding their health. For instance, if heart disease is the number-one killer of women, why are medications and treatment plans often designed for male heart patients? Priest offers questions you need to ask your health care providers, and ways that you can become involved on a personal and political level to work towards a fairer and more accountable system.

Lisa Priest is an award-winning journalist and author of the best-selling Conspiracy of Silence *(made into a CBC-TV movie) and* Women Who Killed. *She currently works as an investigative reporter for the* Globe and Mail. *She lives in Toronto.*

Internet Resources

Online Support and Discussion Groups

Jeannah's Hysterectomy Awareness Web Site
www.hysterectomyawareness.com
Hysterectomy Awareness is a "labour of love" designed for women in search of information regarding hysterectomy, oophorectomy, hormone replacement therapy, natural hormone replacement therapy, and endometriosis. The site includes a special section where women have generously contributed their own hysterectomy experiences, a large collection of Internet resources and pertinent links, Jeannah's own candid account of her hysterectomy experience, journal entries, and compounding pharmacy listings in the United States, Canada, and the United Kingdom.

Sans Uteri Hysterectomy Forum
www.findings.net/sans-uteri.html
More than six hundred thousand women are hysterectomized every year in the United States alone. If you have had a hysterectomy or have been advised to have one, here is where you can find support. Now there is a safe place for women to discuss the many challenges that this surgery brings to their lives and to share ideas. Sans Uteri offers an active Internet mailing list, open to women facing hysterectomy, hysterectomized women, and their significant others. Open communication between hysterectomized women and women considering surgery is the best way to ensure that they make careful and wise decisions about consenting to the removal of their reproductive organs.

Sans Uteri is sponsored by Findings. A donation of US$12 per year is requested. The list owner and moderator is Beth Tiner, 1621 Glyndon Avenue, Venice, CA 90291. Sans Uteri's e-mail address is **findings@findings.net**.

Women's Wellness Network
www.wwn.on.ca

The Women's Wellness Network is an online interactive community dedicated to educating women about wellness. The goal at the Women's Wellness Network is to educate and guide women with the information they require to live a healthy life. The network has many features, including an online Web page of health services and professionals. The directory provides members with a complementary range of both alternative and traditional professionals. The online advisory board consists of local professionals who volunteer their time and expertise. Board members are responsible for the content of a monthly online magazine. Archived articles written by professionals from all over the world provide members with up-to-date information. The online fitness centre is contributed by two separate fitness centres in Toronto; monthly articles and exercise techniques are provided.

84 Abbott Avenue, Toronto, ON M6P 1H6
(416) 766-1956 (tel.); (416) 588-1315 (fax)
E-mail: **support@wwn.on.ca**

Informed Consent

InformedConsent.org Foundation
www.InformedConsent.org

The non-profit InformedConsent.org Foundation was founded by Eileen Marie Wayne, M.D. Its mission is to provide informed consent documents both to take home and keep and to make a permanent part of legal medical records for every medical, surgical, diagnostic, and therapeutic procedure. Dr. Wayne can be contacted by e-mail at **EileenWayneMD@InformedConsent.org**.

Medical Resources

Boston Women's Health Book Collective
www.ourbodiesourselves.org
The Boston Women's Health Book Collective (BWHBC) is a non-profit, public interest women's health education, advocacy, and consulting organization. Beginning in 1970 with the publication of the first edition of *Our Bodies, Ourselves* and continuing for thirty years, the BWHBC has inspired the women's health movement by

- producing a book that makes accurate health and medical information accessible to a broad audience by weaving women's stories into a framework of practical, clearly written text;
- identifying and collaborating with exemplary individuals and organizations that provide services, generate research and policy analysis, and organize for social change; and
- inspiring and empowering women to become engaged in the political aspects of sustaining good health for themselves and their communities.

Judy Norsigian
Executive Director of *Our Bodies, Ourselves for the New Century*
Co-founder of the Boston Women's Health Book Collective
34 Plympton Street, Boston, MA 02118, USA
(617) 451-3666 (direct phone); (617) 451-3664 (fax)
E-mail: **judy@bwhbc.org**

A Friend Indeed (AFI)
www.afriendindeed.ca

A Friend Indeed is the only non-profit and advertisement-free newsletter for women in menopause and mid-life. It is a respected source of understandable and reliable information about the menopausal transition, independent of any vested interests. AFI is published 6 times yearly and distributed to thousands of women across North America.

AFI has provided women with unbiased information about menopause since 1984. We exist solely through the support of our subscriber base.

For over 18 years subscribers have trusted A Friend Indeed to provide them with well-researched, balanced health information and support. We cover a wide range of women's health information in every issue, such as:

- pros and cons of hormone therapy
- perimenopause
- heart disease
- osteoporosis and bone cancer
- breast cancer — prevention and treatment
- complementary medicine
- menopausal weight gain and body image
- suggestions for being careful consumers of health products and the health care system

A Friend Indeed
Main Floor, 419 Graham Avenue, Winnipeg, MB, R3C 0M3 Canada
or
PO Box 260 Pembina, ND, 58271-0260 USA
E-mail: afi@afriendindeed.ca

Medical Breakthroughs — Medical News and Health Information
www.ivanhoe.com

Ivanhoe.com features daily news on the latest advances in medicine.

Launched in January 1996, it was a logical extension of Ivanhoe Broadcast News' syndicated TV series, *Medical Breakthroughs*, that is carried by 150 television stations across the United States. The web site provides viewers with creative, top-quality and thought-provoking news stories that offer the latest breakthroughs in medicine and tips on staying healthy by:

- featuring groundbreaking news in 19 health channels including Breast Cancer, Fertility & Pregnancy, and Women's Health;
- hosting discussion groups led by national medical experts;
- producing a daily e-mail subscription service called "Medical Alerts!" that automatically sends you an e-mail every time Ivanhoe reports a medical development on your topics of interest; and
- offering over 4,500 archived reports for the benefit of those searching for treatments by leading specialists from around the country.

2745 West Fairbanks Avenue, Winter Park, FL 32789
(407) 691-1500 (tel.); (407) 740-5320 (fax)
E-mail: **webdoctor@ivanhoe.com**

Energy Medicine Magazine
www.energymedicineonline.com
Live Your Best Life

Energy Medicine introduces beneficial, safe and healthful information to aid you in living a meaningful life. We feature selected articles, practitioners and authors who support and empower your life choices. We share with you the proven results that doctors, experts and leaders in the field of mind/body medicine have discovered in an easy to read format.

Energy Medicine reminds you of your inherent freedom to choose again. We provide pertinent information that will empower your life, enrich your decisions and heal your relationships. All of us, working in community, toward helping you remember and appreciate that your spirit goes on and that you are not alone.

Wanda Bowring, Publisher
1369 Kingston Avenue, Ottawa, Ontario, Canada, K1Z 8L1
(613) 722-6323 (tel.); (613) 722-2672 (fax)
E-mail: office@energymedicineonline.com

The Ontario Women's Health Council
www.ontariowomenshealthcouncil.on.ca

The Ontario Women's Health Council was established in 1998 by the Minister of Health to act as an advocate and a catalyst for change to improve the health of women in Ontario, Canada, at all stages of life.
The mandate of the Council is:

- to advise the Minister of Health and Long-Term Care and key stake holders on health issues affecting women;
- to advocate for improvements in women's health in Ontario;
- to promote, influence and disseminate research into women's health issues;
- to reach out and empower women across the province to make informed decisions that will contribute to improvements in their health.

Council members would like to hear from you. The interests and concerns of women of Ontario are important to them and will help guide their work and their success.
For more information on the Ontario Women's Health Council, you can e-mail them from their web site, or write them at:

Ontario Women's Health Council Secretariat
880 Bay Street, 2nd Floor, Toronto, Ontario M5S 1Z8
(416) 327-8348 (tel.); (416) 327-3200 (fax)

General Medical Information

Melbourne International Medicine Associate
www.mima.com

WebMD
www.my.webmd.com

HealthScout
www.healthscout.com

Harvard Center for Cancer Prevention, Your Cancer Risk
www.yourcancerrisk.harvard.edu

MayoClinic.com
www.mayohealth.org

American Cancer Society
www.cancer.org

Canadian Cancer Society
www.cancer.ca

Association of Cancer Online Resources
www.acor.org

OncoChat: Online Peer Support for Cancer Survivors, Families, and Friends
www.oncochat.org

Steve Dunn's CancerGuide
www.cancerguide.org

General Drug Information

Clinical Pharmacology Online: Internet Drug Reference
cp.gsm.com/fromcpo.asp

FDA Drug Information
www.fda.gov/cder/drug/default.htm

Informed Drug Guide
www.infomed.org/100drugs

Nurses' PDR Resource Center
www.drugref.com

PDR.net for Physicians
www.pdr.net/physician

PharmWeb
www.PharmWeb.net

Rx List
www.rxlist.com

University of Wisconsin Antibiotic Guidelines
www.medsch.wisc.edu/clinsci/amcg/amcg.html

Adhesions

"Contemporary Adhesion Prevention,"
www.centerforendo.com/news/adhesions/adhesions.htm

Alternatives to Hysterectomy

"Alternative Therapy: The Uterus"
www.wellweb.com/ALTERN/column/uterus.htm

"Why Would a Woman Resist Hysterectomy?" Michael E. Toaff, M.D.,
MSc
www.netreach.net/~hysterectomyedu/whywould.html

Bone Loss

"ESCT: Fosamax Prevents Rapid Bone Loss in Women Who Discontinue HRT"
www.pslgroup.com/dg/fc872.htm

"Postmenopausal Bone Loss Prevented with Low Dose HRT Plus Calcium"
www.pslgroup.com/dg/1020d6.htm

"Calcium and Osteoporosis"
www.health-science.com/calcium.htm

Candida (Yeast Infection)

Books on Candida
howdyneighbor.com/jbayliss/candbook.htm

YEAST-L Mailing List
www.howdyneighbor.com/jbayliss/listinfo.htm
The YEAST-L list is for discussion of Candida allergy and overgrowth, and the sharing of remedies and personal experiences related to yeast problems. While it is meant to be a casual discussion list, people from the medical community are also welcome. To subscribe to the YEAST-L list, send an e-mail to **listserv@maelstrom.stjohns.edu**. The subject line is not important, but in the body of your note you must type "subscribe to YEAST-L" and your name.

Endocrine System

"Endocrine Disrupters Travel Far"
www.innerbody.com/image/endoov.html
"Endocrine System Overview"
www.parksville.net/wellness/1298/liver.htm

Endometriosis

Reproductive Specialty Center, "Endometriosis: Update on Endometriosis Treatment by Laparoscopy"
www.reproductivecenter.com

Fibromyalgia

Information on fibromyalgia developing after hysterectomy
www.marysherbs.com/heal-fbm.htm

Miryam Ehrlich Williamson's site on improving quality of life for fibromyalgia sufferers
www.mwilliamson.com

Hormones

Cenestin
www.oxford.net/~tishy/cenestin.html
"Comparative Measurements of Serum Estriol, Estradiol, and Estrone in Non-pregnant Premenopausal Women: A Preliminary Investigation"
www.thorne.com/altmedrev/estriol-ab4-4.html

Conjugated Estrogens
www.rxlist.com/cgi/generic/conest.htm

DHEA (how you can relieve depression with DHEA)
www.lef.org/featured-articles/dheaupdate1.html

DHEA
www.ceri.com/dhea.htm

Estradiol
www.aeron.com/estradiol.htm; highlandpharmacy.com/Estradiol.htm

Estriol
www.aeron.com/estriol.htm;
www.highlandpharmacy.com/Estriol.htm

Estrogen Dominance
www.health-science.com/estrodom.htm

Estrogen Replacement Therapy
ffirx.com/information_center/femscript/estrogen_replacement_therapy/
index.html

Estrone
www.highlandpharmacy.com/Estrone.htm

"The Little Hormone Book"
www.naturalhormoneclinic.com

Osteoporosis and Natural Progesterone
www.health-science.com/osteo.htm

Progesterone
www.aeron.com/progesterone.htm

"Prometrium: Progestins & Progesterone"
www.rxmed.com/rxmed/a.home.html
(Click on "Pharmaceutical Information," "P," then "Prometrium.")

Testosterone
www.naturalhealthworld.com/articles/testost.html;
www.whas.com.au/testosterone.shtml

Hormone Replacement Therapy and Natural HRT

"Answering the Natural Question"
www.mountainviewpharmacy.com/natural2.html

"Benefits of NHRT"
www.troubleshooter.com/data/columns/naturalhormonereplacement.htm

*"Combination HRT Increases Breast Cancer Risk, NOT If You Are
Taking Natural Hormones"*
www.debfnp.com/hormones.html

"Common Myths About HRT"
www.medicalcenter.net/hormone_replacement_therapy_myth_6.htm

"Contemporary Pharmaceutical Compounding"
hometown.aol.com/mefrancom/contcmpd.html

"Dangers and Risks of HRT: Letter to Patients & Physicians Regarding Increased Risk of Cancer and Hormones"
www.goodliferx.com/letter.htm

"Hormone Replacement Therapy"
age-reversing-miracle.com/hrt.html

"Natural Bio-Identical Hormone Replacement"
www.cairx.com/natural.htm

"Natural Hormones"
www.naturalhormoneclinic.com/

"Natural Hormone Replacement: Overview"
www.surgimenopause.com/NoFrames/nhrt_main.html

"Natural Hormone Replacement Reduces Cancer Risk"
www.kirlian.org/life_enhancement_products/nhr.html

"Natural Hormone Replacement Therapy"
keynutritionrx.com/hrt.htm

"Natural Hormone Replacement Therapy"
www.aeron.com/newsletter_.htm

"Premarin: The Politics of Pharmaceuticals," Judy Mann (Washington Post)
www.sherryart.com/women/estrogens/jmann.html

"Talking to Your Doctor About HRT"
www.aeron.com/new_page_21.htm

"What Are Natural or Bio-Identical Hormones?"
www.kdlk.com/brochure_page.cfm?BusinessID=94

Hysterectomy and Menopause

"Menopause Information" (June 1999)
www.pslgroup.com/menopause.htm

"Vivelle-Dot Available in the US for Menopause Symptoms" (June 1999)
www.pslgroup.com/dg/fc87a.htm

"Oophorectomy or Hysterectomy After Age 40? A Practice That Does Not Withstand Scrutiny," Winnifred B. Cutler, Ph.D.
athena-inst.com/oophorectomy.html

"Postmenopausal Bone Loss Prevented with Low Dose HRT Plus Calcium"
www.pslgroup.com/dg/1020d6.htm

Sexuality

"Abdominal Hysterectomy: Trends, Analysis, and Sexual Function?"
www.obgyn.net/ah/articles/special_5-99.htm

"The Hidden Power of Body Odors: Studies find that male pheromones are good for women's health," John Lea *(Time, December 1, 1986)*
www.athena-inst.com/mediaarticles/time12186.html

"Hysterectomy and Sexual Orgasm"
www.thriveonline.aol.com/health/experts/bill/bill.07-21-99.html

"More on Sex After Hysterectomy"
www.drweil.com/drw/app/cda/drw_cda.php
(Type "hysterectomy" into the site's search function to get to this article.)

"Is Orgasm Gone After Hysterectomy?"
www.wdxcyber.com/m2hyst.htm#m09

"Progesterone and Libido"
www.sheld.com/lifeflo/1libido.html

"Testosterone Patch Effective for Diminished Sexual Function in Surgically Menopausal Women"
www.pslgroup.com/dg/107bc2.htm

Tubal Ligation

"Tubal Ligation — Aftereffects"
www.tubal.org

Weight Gain After Hysterectomy

"HRT and Weight Gain"
www.askthedietitian.com/hormones.html

"Weight Gain and Adrenal Hormones"
www.gsdl.com/assessments/finddisease/weight/adrenal_hormones.html

"Thyroid Function and Hormones"
members.tripod.com/~HealthInfo/

"Weight Cycling May Be Linked to Hysterectomy"
www.goddessdiet.com/menopause.htm

"Low Hormone Levels May Encourage Weight Gain"
www.lubbockonline.com/news/013197/low.htm

"Weight Gain After a Hysterectomy"
www.estronaut.com/a/hysterectomy_weight.htm

Clinics, Support Groups, Organizations, and Advocacy Groups

Canadian Premenstrual Syndrome Clinic/Clinique du Syndrome Prémenstruel
Louise Laberge, M.D., and Richard Bergeron, M.D.
Pierre-Janet Hospital Centre
20 Pharand Street, Hull, QC J9A 1K7
Tel: (819) 776-8027, Fax: (819) 771-4849

Women who suffer from PMS can contact this clinic for help. Doctors Laberge and Bergeron offer help and advice on how to alleviate PMS symptoms through lifestyle changes, good nutrition, and vitamin or other supplemental therapies.

HERS Foundation (Hysterectomy Educational Resources and Services)
Nora Coffey, President
422 Bryn Mawr Avenue, Bala Cynwood, PA 19004
Tel: (610) 667-7757, Fax: (610) 667-8096
Web site: **www.hersfoundation.com**

Ontario Women's Health Network
180 Dundas Street West, Toronto, ON M5G 1Z8
Toll-free: 1-877-860-4545, Tel: (416) 408-4840
Web site: **www.owhn.on.ca**

Endometriosis Association
P.O. Box 921187, Milwaukee, WI 53202
Toll-free: 1-800-992-3636
E-mail: **endo@endometriosisassn.org**

EA is a self-help organization for women with endometriosis, and for others interested in offering mutual support and help to those afflicted by endometriosis, educating the public and medical community about the disease and promoting research related to it. The organization has published two books, *Overcoming Endometriosis* and *The Endometriosis Sourcebook*.

Ontario Fibromyalgia Association
Based in Ontario, Canada, the OFA's contact person is Lynn Cooper.
Toll-free: 1-800-321-1433

Interstitial Cystitis (Urinary Urgency and Frequency)
For this free information kit about interstitial cystitis, including a video-cassette, contact:
Alza Canada, 2900 John Street, Unit 1, Markham, ON L3R 5G3
Toll-free: 1-800-668-3535, Tel: (905) 475-9777, Fax: (905) 475-2996

Voices on Health-Care Concerns and Accountability: Support, Advocacy, Information (VoHCA)
P.O. Box 27018, Gardiners Post Office, Kingston, ON K7M 8W4
Tel: (613) 389-5599, Fax: (613) 389-8036

VoHCA acts as the voice of patients in Canada to ensure that the health care system meets their needs. The purpose of VoHCA is to act nationally as a patient advocacy group by

- providing support on a local level for patients and their families who have had, or who are having, problems with the health care system;
- working with government and health care providers to make the system accountable to the public; and
- providing current information to allow patients to make informed choices about their health care system.

Salivary Testing

Salivary testing is the most accurate procedure for determining a hysterectomized woman's hormonal levels. Laboratories in Canada do not perform this test, but it can be done by the following U.S. laboratories:

Aeron Life Cycles
1933 Davis Street, Suite 310, San Leandro, CA 94577-9826
Toll-free: 1-800-631-7900

You can obtain a testing tube by mail, by writing, or by calling Aeron Life Cycles. Your doctor can also order one for you. At present, the cost to Canadian women for salivary testing is US$140.

Diagnos-Techs, Inc.
The contact person for this Seattle, Washington, firm is David Zava, at (425) 251-0596.

ZRT Laboratory
12505 NW Cornell Road, Portland, OR 97229
Tel: (503) 469-0741, Fax: (503) 469-1305
E-mail: **dtzava@aol.com**

Compounding Pharmacies

International Academy of Compounding Pharmacists
P.O. Box 1365, Sugar Land, TX 77487
Toll-free: 1-800-927-4227, Tel: (713) 933-8400, Fax: (281) 495-0602
Web site: **www.iacprx.org**

Contact the Academy to locate a compounding pharmacy in your area. They will provide the names and addresses of compounding pharmacists in the United States, Canada, and Australia.

La pharmacie du Medical Arts: A natural pharmacy
Don Pearson and Mel Alter, Compounding Pharmacists
5025 Sherbrooke Street West, Westmount, QC H4A 1S9
Tel: (514) 484-2222, Fax: (514) 484-2205
E-mail: **rxp@videotron.ca**

Nutri-Chem Compounding Pharmacy: Bridging the gap between nutrition and chemistry
1303 Richmond Road, Ottawa, ON K2B 7Y4
Tel: (613) 820-4200, Fax: (613) 829-2226
Web site: **www.nutrichem.com**

York Downs Pharmacy
3910 Bathurst Street, Toronto, ON M3H 3N8
Toll-free: 1-800-564-5020, Tel: (416) 633-2244, Fax: (416) 633-3400

This is a compounding pharmacy that integrates complementary medicine with mainstream medicine.

Village Pharmacy and Health Food Store

225 Lakeshore Road East, Mississauga, ON L5G 1G8

Toll-free: 1-800-268-5229, Tel: (905) 278-7237, Fax: (905) 278-3363

This natural compounding pharmacy offers free delivery ($30 minimum order) anywhere in Canada. They make natural estrogen and progesterone and will formulate an anti-inflammatory to be absorbed through your skin and applied to your joints where needed.

Pete Hueseman, R. Ph., P.D.
Bellevue Pharmacy Solutions

1034 So. Brentwood Blvd., Suite 102, St. Louis, MO 63117

(800) 728-0288 (toll free), or (314) 727-8787 (tel.)

(800) 458-9182 (toll free fax), or (314) 727-2830 (fax)

E-mail: ConsultPh@aol.com

www.bpharmacysolutions.com

Pete Hueseman has helped many hysterectomized women with useful information and service. He has a lot of expertise in the area of bio identical hormones and provides caring advice. Available through his pharmacy are: sublinguals, caps, caps in "oil", suppos, creams and gels. He accepts insurances, including CIGNA, and provides many delivery options.

Questions to Ask Your Doctor

When Hysterectomy, Oophorectomy, or Other Pelvic Surgery Is Recommended

1. Why have you recommended a hysterectomy?

2. I understand that hysterectomy is necessary only if I have cancer. If I do not have cancer, why should I agree to have my reproductive organs removed?

3. Will any of my symptoms subside once I enter natural menopause?

4. Have all the proper diagnostic tests — for example, laparoscopy, blood tests, ultrasound, X-ray, or MRI — been done to determine that I have the condition for which you're recommending hysterectomy?

5. Are there other, less invasive treatment options for me to consider? If so, what are they? What are the risks involved with these options?

6. If you are recommending hysterectomy to treat fibroid tumours, are you qualified to perform a myomectomy instead? What are the benefits and risks of myomectomy versus hysterectomy?

7. What are the surgical risks of hysterectomy?

8. What can I expect to happen if I don't have surgery?

9. What reproductive organs do you propose to remove in this operation (uterus, ovaries, Fallopian tubes, cervix)?

10. What surgical procedure do you propose to use to perform my hysterectomy: abdominal, vaginal, or laparoscopy-assisted vaginal? Why?

11. What type of incision will you make? Do you make Pfannensteil (bikini-line) incisions? If not, why not?

12. If my ovaries are removed, will I be able to maintain a healthy libido?

13. If you are proposing to remove my ovaries to avoid ovarian cancer, what risk factors do I have for ovarian cancer that suggest these vital organs should be removed prophylactically?

14. If you are proposing to remove my cervix, why have you chosen to do so?

15. If my cervix is removed, will my vagina be shortened? Will you use the "Worrelling" technique to preserve its length?

16. If my vagina is shortened, will sexual intercourse be possible? Will full penetration be possible?

17. If my uterus is removed, will its removal affect orgasm? Why or why not?

18. Many nerves will have to be cut to remove my reproductive organs. How will this affect my sexual responses? Will orgasm and sexual pleasure be the same?

19. Are you qualified to perform a nerve-sparing hysterectomy?

20. Who will perform my hysterectomy — you, another gynecological surgeon, or a resident-in-training?

21. Who will be the anesthesiologist?

22. Can I have a referral to see the anesthesiologist? I would like to ask about the risks involved with the anesthetics that will be used during surgery, and to discuss my preferred choice of anesthetic.

23. Can I make arrangements to have my hysterectomy videotaped?

24. What are all the possible side effects of hysterectomy and/or oophorectomy? What are the best- and worst-case scenarios?

25. Will I be going into menopause after this surgery?

26. What's the difference between natural and surgical menopause?

27. If my menopause is surgically induced, will any symptoms I may experience be more severe than those experienced by women who enter menopause naturally?

28. How do you propose to treat any potential side effects from early menopause?

29. If I do experience any side effects from hysterectomy, how long will they last?

30. Can hormone replacement therapy provide adequate relief from all the side effects I may experience following a hysterectomy?

31. What are the side effects of hormone replacement therapy?

32. Will you be monitoring my progress on hormone replacement therapy?

33. If my body reacts negatively to hormone replacement therapy, how will I be able to control any side effects I may experience, and how will you be able to help me if this happens?

34. Are you familiar with natural hormone replacement therapy? Would you be willing to prescribe it if I asked you to?

35. Can hormone replacement therapy effectively restore lost libido? Why or why not?

36. Could I have the names and telephone numbers of other women on whom you have performed a hysterectomy?

37. How long will it take me to recover from hysterectomy?

38. How long before I can resume sexual activity?

39. If sex becomes painful and difficult, what would be your course of treatment to resolve this problem?

Medical Terminology

abdominal myomectomy: a surgical procedure to remove fibroids. Sometimes the procedure is performed by making a bikini-line or midline incision in the abdominal area. In this procedure, a woman's uterus and ovaries remain intact.

acupuncture: the Chinese medical practice of inserting needles at specific points on the body to relieve pain. This method of treatment is often relied upon as a preventive measure.

acute: used to describe a sharp pain or a problem accompanied by severe symptoms but of short duration.

adhesion: Following any type of abdominal surgery, inner tissue surfaces may join to form adhesions. Fibrous scar tissue normally forms around an incision when the body is healing. Sometimes the scar tissue may cling to adjoining organs, possibly resulting in pain. If pain persists, further surgery may be required to either smooth out or remove the adhesions.

anal: related to the anus.

analgesic: a drug capable of reducing sensibility to pain.

anemia: a blood deficiency, usually of hemoglobin, that can result in pallor and weakness, often caused by excessive blood loss.

anesthesia: insensibility to pain induced by a drug administered prior to an operation.

anesthetic: a drug normally administered by an anesthetist to help patients relax prior to a surgical procedure and to achieve insensibility to pain.

anesthetist: a medical doctor who specializes in the administration of anesthetics.

antidepressant: a drug normally prescribed to patients who suffer from depression or an anxiety disorder. Many of these drugs (for example, Paxil, Zoloft, and Prozac) can have serious side effects, including loss of libido.

anus: the excretory opening at the end of the digestive tract.

appendectomy: a surgical procedure to remove a patient's appendix.

artery: a vessel that carries blood from the heart to other parts of the body.

asexual: not sexually active; having no desire to have sex.

asymptomatic: showing or causing no symptoms.

atrophy: a shrinking or wasting.

benign growth: a non-cancerous growth that is not a threat to health.

beta-blocker: a type of heart drug.

biochemistry: the science of chemical reactions or the chemistry of living organisms.

biopsy: an examination of body tissue to determine whether it is cancerous.

bladder: an organ that resembles a sac, whose main function is to act as a receptacle for urine manufactured by the kidneys.

bowel: another name for the large intestine.

Caesarean section: a surgical procedure in which a baby is delivered through incisions made in the abdominal wall and uterus.

Candida: a parasitic yeast fungus that can appear in the mouth, skin, intestine, or vagina, resulting in infection.

candidiasis: an infectious condition of the skin, mouth, respiratory tract, or vagina caused by the Candida fungi.

cardiovascular: relating to the heart and its blood vessels.

carpal tunnel syndrome: a condition causing pain and loss of sensation in the fingers and hand, caused by compression of the meridian nerve in the wrist.

castration: surgical removal or destruction of a woman's ovaries or a man's testes.

catheter: a flexible tube inserted into a body canal or cavity to either remove or inject fluids.

cauterization: a procedure in which a hot iron, electrical current, or a chemical agent is used to burn and destroy tissue.

cervix: the narrow lower end of the uterus where it opens into the vagina.

chemotherapy: the use of chemical agents (medication) to control disease.

chronic: describes symptoms or a condition that progresses slowly and continues over a long period of time.

clitoris: the small erectile organ situated in the frontal part of the vulva.

clotting: a process in which blood forms into thick masses, interfering with the flow of normal blood.

coagulation: the process by which blood or liquid forms into a clot.

colon: the large intestine (bowel).

coronary vasoconstriction: a decrease of the caliber of the blood vessels of the heart.

cyclic: occurring in cycles.

cyst: a closed sac; an abnormal growth surrounded by a membrane. Though most cysts do not pose an immediate threat, they can lead to malignancy.

cystitis: inflammation of the urinary bladder.

cystogram: a diagnostic record made during cystography.

cystography: X-ray of the urinary tract. A substance is injected into the bladder and the cystography is done as the patient urinates.

cystoscopy: examination of the bladder using a cystoscope.

D&C: *see* dilation and curettage.

depression: a mental disorder characterized by extreme sadness and despair that can affect one's appetite, sleep pattern, and ability to function.

dermatologist: a medical doctor specializing in the treatment of skin disorders.

diagnosis: complete understanding of an illness obtained by testing and examination of the patient.

dilation and curettage (D&C): a procedure in which various instruments are used to stretch the vagina and enter the cervix. An instrument called a curette is then inserted so that the surgeon can scrape away the lining of the uterus.

distension: the state of being abnormally enlarged.

diuretic: an agent that produces an increased flow of urine.

dysmenorrhea: painful menses (menstruation), usually accompanied by cramps.

dyspareunia: pain with intercourse.

edema: abnormal accumulation of fluid in the tissues or in a body cavity surrounded by a membrane.

embolization: a procedure that involves injection of a substance into a blood vessel in order to obstruct or cut off the flow of blood to a specific area or growth.

endocrine glands: glands that secrete hormones in the body. They include the hypothalamus, thyroid, pituitary, and adrenal glands, the ovaries in women, and the testes in men.

endocrinologist: a medical doctor who specializes in the study of endocrine glands and their related disorders.

endometrial: related to the endometrium, the lining of the uterus.

endometrioma: endometrial tissue growing in an ovary, also known as a "chocolate" cyst.

endometriosis: a condition in which endometrial tissue grows outside the uterus and moves into other areas of the pelvic cavity or body. It can lead to severe pain, abnormal bleeding, and possible infertility.

endometrium: the lining of the uterus.

enema: the introduction of liquid into the rectum to cleanse the intestine of fecal matter.

epidural: the strongest of three membranes surrounding the brain and the spinal cord.

epidural anesthesia: an injection of anesthetic directly into the epidural.

ERT: *see* estrogen replacement therapy.

estrogen: a sex hormone comprising three types of estrogen: estradiol, estrone, and estriol. Estrogen hormones are secreted mainly by the ovaries in women and the testes in men. The adrenal glands also produce estrogens, although in smaller amounts.

estrogen replacement therapy (ERT): a drug treatment for postmenopausal women that comes in many forms, most commonly the drug Premarin. ERT can also be prescribed as a transdermal cream or gel, or in the form of a patch. This therapy is intended to mimic what a woman's body used to produce more efficiently before surgical or natural menopause. There are many side effects to long-term use of ERT, so read the label, and insist on careful monitoring by your family physician.

exploratory surgery: surgery to investigate a patient's complaint or problem in order to obtain an accurate diagnosis.

Fallopian tube: one of two tubes located on each side of the uterus whose principal function is to carry eggs from the ovaries to the uterus.

fibrocystic: related to the growth of fibrous tissue and cysts.

fibroid: a benign tumour or growth of muscle tissue in the uterus.

fibromyalgia: a rheumatic disorder that causes pain and stiffness of the muscles and joints.

fibrous: containing fibres.

flush: *see* hot flash.

follicle: a small sac or cavity.

follicle-stimulating hormone (FSH): a hormone produced by the pituitary gland whose main function is to stimulate growth of the egg-containing follicles in the ovaries.

gallbladder: a sac shaped like a pear, located below the liver, that stores bile for subsequent delivery to the small intestine.

gastric: related to the stomach.

gastrointestinal (GI): related to the stomach and intestines.

genitalia: the sex organs of the reproductive system.

GI: *see* gastrointestinal.

GnRH: gonadotropin-releasing hormone, a hormone that stimulates the gonads.

gonad: a reproductive or sex gland; the ovaries in women and the testes in men.

gynecologist: a medical doctor who specializes in the medical and surgical treatment of disorders specific to women.

gynecology: the medical specialty that deals with the study and treatment of disorders specific to women.

hemorrhage: abundant discharge of blood from blood vessels.

hernia: a bulge or protrusion of part of an organ or body tissue.

homeopathy: a form of medical treatment that uses very small, diluted doses of substances that would produce symptoms similar to those of the disease being treated when used at full strength.

hormone: a chemical messenger produced by the glands of the body's endocrine system. Hormones travel through the bloodstream to stimulate and control many bodily functions, for example, growth, reproduction, sexual attributes, libido, and some mental conditions and personality traits.

hormone replacement therapy (HRT): a drug treatment prescribed for postmenopausal women that uses one or more hormones to mimic what the body used to do more efficiently before surgical or natural menopause. HRT comes in many forms, for example, tablets, transdermal creams or gels, or patches. There are many side effects to long-term use of HRT, so read the label, and insist on careful monitoring by your family physician.

hot flash (flush): a surge of heat from the middle area of the body to the top of the head, sometimes causing redness of the face and neck; the most common aftereffect of surgical and natural menopause. It is caused by diminished hormone levels and is normally accompanied by an increased heartbeat. The flush eventually reaches a peak point, after which there will be a slow release of the intense heat.

HRT: *see* hormone replacement therapy.

hydronephrosis: abnormal enlargement of the kidney caused by a blockage of the urinary tract.

hyper-: excessive.

hypersensitivity: an exaggerated reaction of the body to a stimulus.

hypertension: high blood pressure.

hypnosis: the placing of a person into a trance by a specialist in hypnotherapy.

hypo-: abnormally deficient.

hypochondriac: a person overly preoccupied by his/her health; one who imagines symptoms of serious illness.

hysterectomy: a surgical procedure involving the total or sometimes partial removal of a woman's uterus (womb).

hystero-oophorectomy: a surgical procedure involving removal of a woman's uterus and both ovaries.

hysterosalpingo-oophorectomy: a surgical procedure involving removal of a woman's uterus, ovaries, and Fallopian tubes.

hysteroscopic myomectomy: a surgical procedure involving removal of fibroids through the vaginal canal by inserting a hysteroscope, an instrument resembling a telescope, into the vagina, through the cervix, and into the uterus.

IC: *see* interstitial cystitis.

ileus: an obstruction of the bowel (intestine).

implant: something natural or artificial inserted into the body.

incontinence: failure of the body to restrain or control the release of urine or feces.

insomnia: a sleep disorder that prevents one from falling asleep or from getting a complete night's sleep.

internist: a medical doctor who specializes in diagnosis of internal disorders and in treatment with drugs.

interstitial: within or between organs or tissue.

interstitial cystitis (IC): a condition that results in excessive urgency and frequency of urination. Sufferers may experience pain, suprapubic discomfort, and excessive urination at night.

intestinal: related to the intestine.

intravenous (IV): situated, performed, or occurring within a vein.

IVP: intravenous pyelogram. A pyelogram is the film produced by pyelography, an X-ray test of the kidney and ureter conducted by injecting a liquid (or dye) intravenously.

LAH: *see* laparoscopy-assisted vaginal hysterectomy.

laminectomy: a surgical procedure involving removal of an arch-shaped structure in the vertebra (a bony segment of the spinal cord).

laparoscope: a surgical instrument used to examine the organs in the abdominal cavity or to guide other surgical procedures performed in the abdomen.

laparoscopic myolysis: a surgical procedure performed to stop a fibroid from growing, involving insertion of surgical instruments into an abdominal incision, usually at the navel. The instruments release a high-frequency electrical current at the base of a fibroid in order to cut off its blood supply. The fibroid is not surgically removed, but without a blood supply, it will shrink and eventually die.

laparoscopic myomectomy: a surgical procedure involving the removal of fibroids using a laparoscope, through incisions made in the navel and at other sites in the abdominal area.

laparoscopy: a surgical procedure for examination of the organs in the abdominal cavity.

laparoscopy-assisted vaginal hysterectomy (LAVH): a surgical procedure involving removal of a woman's uterus through the vagina, using a laparoscope. The cervix, Fallopian tubes, and ovaries may or may not be removed also.

laparotomy: a surgical procedure involving a large abdominal incision so that the organs can be examined.

LAVH: *see* laparoscopy-assisted vaginal hysterectomy.

lesion: damage to a body part caused by disease or possibly trauma.

lethargic: affected by lethargy.

lethargy: a condition of abnormal drowsiness, sluggishness, or indifference.

libido: the sex drive; sexual desire.

lidocaine: a drug used as a local anesthetic.

LSH: laparoscopic supracervical hysterectomy, a surgical procedure involving the removal of the uterus, leaving all or part of the cervix intact.

lymph node: a collection of stationary lymph cells. Lymph nodes are part of the immune system, and are found all over the body.

magnetic resonance imaging (MRI): an imaging technique that uses magnetic waves to examine body tissues.

malignant: cancerous; having the capability to invade and spread to other body organs.

mammogram: an X-ray of the breast.

mastalgia: breast pain.

menopause: cessation of the menstrual flow that normally occurs in women between the ages of forty-five and fifty-five.

menses: the monthly discharge of blood that occurs in menstruation; a woman's period.

menstrual: related to menstruation.

menstrual cycle: the buildup and periodic shedding of the lining of the uterus that occurs on average every twenty-eight days, with a discharge that lasts approximately five days.

MRI: *see* magnetic resonance imaging.

myoma: a benign tumour of muscle tissue.

myomectomy: a surgical procedure involving excision (cutting out) of a myoma.

myometrium: the muscular lining of the uterus.

narcotic: an addictive drug that dulls the senses when taken in small doses and induces stupor and profound sleep in large doses.

NHRT: natural hormone replacement therapy, referring to bio-identical hormones for the relief of menopausal symptoms.

obstetrics: the medical specialty dealing with pregnancy, labour, and the delivery of babies.

oncologist: a medical doctor who specializes in the study and treatment of cancer.

oncology: the medical specialty dealing with the study and treatment of cancer.

oophorectomy: a surgical procedure involving removal of one or both ovaries, also known as ovariectomy.

OR: operating room.

orgasm: the climax of sexual excitement.

osteoporosis: a condition resulting in decreased bone density.

ovarian: related to the ovary.

ovariectomy: *see* oophorectomy.

ovary: one of two sex glands in the female abdomen that produces eggs and sex hormones.

ovum: an egg ready to be fertilized and capable of developing into a human being (plural: ova).

Pap test: short for Papanicolaou test or smear, a test used to detect cancer of the uterus and cervix.

pathology: the medical specialty that deals with the study of disease and its causes and effects.

PCA: patient-controlled analgesic, often an intravenous morphine pump, that provides pain control on demand.

pelvic: related to the pelvis or the hip region.

perimenopause: the period of time, usually several years, leading up to natural menopause.

physiology: the science that deals with the activities and functions of living organisms and the physical and chemical processes involved.

PID: pelvic inflammatory disease, a disease of the female pelvic organs, including the Fallopian tubes, uterus, ovaries, and cervix.

PMS: *see* premenstrual syndrome.

polycystic: involving more than one cyst.

post-menopause: the period following menopause (the complete cessation of menstruation).

post-operative care: care of the patient after a surgical operation.

post-traumatic: occurring after a trauma or injury.

post-traumatic stress disorder: an anxiety or psychological disorder that occurs after experiencing an intensely stressful event.

premenstrual: directly preceding menstruation.

premenstrual syndrome (PMS): symptoms occurring immediately before menstruation, which tend to vary from woman to woman, and can include irritability, abrupt mood swings, fatigue, insomnia, anxiety, depression, and pelvic pain.

progesterone: a sex steroid hormone produced by the ovary.

prolapse: downward displacement or slippage of a body part.

prophylactic: used to protect against disease.

pyelogram: the record of the pyelographic X-ray test.

pyelography: an X-ray test of the kidney and ureter that involves injection of a substance through the ureter or into a vein.

pyelonephritis: an inflammatory condition of the kidney and renal pelvis.

quadrant: a quarter-section of a body part.

radical hysterectomy: a surgical procedure involving removal of a woman's uterus, cervix, ovaries, Fallopian tubes, lymph nodes, and lymph channels, normally reserved for the treatment of cancer.

radiologist: a medical doctor who specializes in the use of X-rays to diagnose illness.

rectum: the end of the colon (large intestine) that brings body wastes to the anus.

replacement therapy: the treatment of hormones or blood to replace what is lacking in the body.

retractor: a surgical instrument used to hold back tissues or the edges of a wound.

rheumatologist: a medical doctor who specializes in the treatment of diseases of the joints and muscles.

rheumatology: the medical specialty dealing with joint and muscle diseases.

rhinoplasty: plastic surgery performed on the nose.

sacral: related to the sacrum.

sacrum: the triangular bone located at the base of the spine.

scan: examination of a body organ by using a sensing device capable of transmitting its findings electronically; also, the resulting image or photograph.

scar tissue: body tissue that forms a scar at the site of a wound or injury.

sexual dysfunction: sexual disorder such as loss of libido, poor sexual response, and loss of orgasm caused by physical or psychological changes or possibly nerve damage from a surgical procedure such as hysterectomy.

shingles: an acute disease or inflammation caused by herpes zoster, the virus that also causes chicken pox.

supracervical hysterectomy: a surgical procedure involving removal of a woman's uterus without removing the cervix.

suprapubic: above the pubic hairline.

symptom: a problem observed by a patient or physician that may indicate a disease or disorder.

TAH: *see* total abdominal hysterectomy.

TAHBSO: *see* total abdominal hysterectomy and bilateral salpingo-oophorectomy.

testis: the testicle, one of the pair of male reproductive organs, or gonads (plural: testes).

testosterone: a sex hormone produced by the testes and, in small amounts, by the ovaries and adrenal glands. Testosterone is mainly responsible for development of male secondary sex characteristics and maintenance of a healthy libido.

thyroid gland: the large, butterfly-shaped endocrine gland located at the base of the neck. The main functions of the hormones produced by the thyroid gland are to maintain normal growth and regulate metabolism.

tissue: groups of similar cells working together to perform a specific job in the body.

total abdominal hysterectomy and bilateral salpingo-oophorectomy (TAHBSO): a surgical procedure involving removal of a woman's uterus, cervix, Fallopian tubes, and ovaries.

total abdominal hysterectomy (TAH): a surgical procedure involving removal of a woman's uterus and cervix through an incision in the abdomen.

total vaginal hysterectomy (TVH): a surgical procedure involving removal of a woman's uterus and cervix through the vagina, with or without a bilateral salpingo-oophorectomy.

transdermal: through the skin; describes treatments administered in the form of creams, gels, or patches.

transvaginal: through the vagina, as in a laparoscopy.

tubal ligation: a surgical procedure to tie off the Fallopian tubes to prevent any ova in the ovaries from reaching the uterus, used as a method of female sterilization.

tumour: a benign or malignant mass of tissue.

TVH: *see* total vaginal hysterectomy.

UAE: *see* uterine artery embolization.

ultrasound: a diagnostic method used to detect abnormalities by beaming high-frequency sound waves into the body.

ureter: the tube that carries urine from the kidney to the bladder.

urethra: the tube that carries urine from the bladder to the outside of the body.

urinary: related to urine.

urinary bladder: the sac that serves as a receptacle for urine from the kidneys before it is released through the urethra out of the body.

urologist: a medical doctor who specializes in urology.

urology: the medical specialty that deals with the study and treatment of the urinary system and the male reproductive tract.

USO: unilateral salpingo-oophorectomy, surgical removal of one ovary.

uterine: related to the uterus.

uterine artery embolization (UAE): a non-surgical procedure to block the blood supply to uterine fibroids, involving injection of particles through a catheter inserted into an artery and then into the uterus. This procedure is performed by an interventional radiologist and takes approximately one hour.

uterus: the pear-shaped, muscular female organ often referred to as the womb, which during pregnancy holds and nourishes the developing fetus.

UTI: urinary tract infection, an infection of the bladder and/or ureter.

vagina: the muscular canal extending from the cervix to the vulva.

vaginal: related to the vagina.

varicose veins: veins that are swollen and knotted because of weaknesses in their walls, often resulting in poor blood flow.

vascular: related to blood vessels.

vertigo: dizziness.

voiding: urination.

vulva: the external genital organs of the female.

Worrelling: a surgical technique to preserve the length of the vagina at hysterectomy. Devised by Dr. Worrell, this technique should be used to carefully peel the vagina away from the cervix, thus avoiding any unnecessary shortening of the vaginal canal that could result in pain with intercourse.

BOOK ORDER FORM

(please check at your local bookstore before using this form)

SHIP TO:

_____
Your Name and Title

_____
Name of Organization (if applicable)

_____

_____
Street Address

City: _____ State: _____ Zip: _____

Telephone: _____

Fax: _____

E-Mail: _____

Please ship _____ copy/copies of **Misinformed Consent.**

I've enclosed $16.95 per copy for copies. $ _____

NJ orders ONLY add 6% sales tax if required ($1.02 per copy) $ _____

Shipping: Add $5.00 for the first copy and

$1.00 for each additional copy $ _____

TOTAL $ _____

A check/money order made payable to Next Decade, Inc.

for $ _____ is enclosed.

Credit Card Payments: ❏ Visa ▬▬   ❏ Mastercard ◉◉

Credit Card # _____ Expiration Date: _____

Name on Card: _____

Signature: _____

Mail to: Next Decade, Inc.
            39 Old Farmstead Road
            Chester, NJ 07930
            Telephone (908) 879-6625 * Fax (908) 879 –2920
            Email: info@nextdecade.com